Getting Started in
Health Research

Getting Started in Health Research

David Bowers
Leeds Institute of Health Sciences
University of Leeds
UK

Allan House
Leeds Institute of Health Sciences
University of Leeds
UK

David Owens
Leeds Institute of Health Sciences
University of Leeds
UK

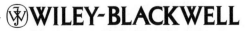

WILEY-BLACKWELL

A John Wiley & Sons, Ltd., Publication

BMJ|Books

Library of Congress Cataloging-in-Publication Data

Bowers, David, 1938–
   Getting started in health research / David Bowers, Allan House, David Owens.
      p. ; cm.
   Includes bibliographical references and index.
   ISBN 978-1-4051-9148-7 (pbk. : alk. paper)
   1. Medicine–Research.   2. Biology–Research.   I. House, Allan.   II. Owens, David, Dr.   III. Title.
   [DNLM: 1. Biomedical Research–methods. W 20.5]
   R852.B69 2011
   610.72–dc22

                                                                        2011002193

A catalogue record for this book is available from the British Library.

This book is published in the following electronic formats: Wiley Online Library 9781444341300

Set in 10/12pt Times Roman by Aptara® Inc., New Delhi, India
Printed and bound in Singapore by Fabulous Printers Pte Ltd

1   2011

Contents

Preface

This book is aimed mainly at those healthcare professionals who want to do some research but have little or no previous research experience – and don't really know where or how to start. If you are decided on your particular research idea this book will be of very great help. We describe all the procedures that are necessary to achieve a successful outcome, and we cover both *quantitative* and *qualitative* research projects.

Why might you want to do some research?

- Because you think it will help your professional (and personal) development;
- Because you want to know the answer to a question related to your professional practice or experience – curiosity;
- Because you have been told to or it is expected of you;
- Because of peer pressure.

Of course there may be other ways to promote your career prospects or to keep up with your peers, doing research is not an easy option and unless you have a strong motivation to do it, it is probably best to find an alternative.

We will take you through the whole research experience, step by step, from the very beginning when that question first pops into your head, 'I wonder why . . . ?', or 'I wonder if . . . ?', to the very end – writing up your idea for publication in a journal, as a paper to be read at a conference, or for submission as part of a thesis or dissertation. The book will provide you with a map of your research journey, telling you what you should be doing at each stage of the process, so that you don't overlook something crucial until it's too late.

As you will see, we have illustrated the various stages of the research process with a blow-by-blow account of the questions, tasks, and potential difficulties of two (fictitious) new researchers, Dinesh (a nurse) and Anna (a general practitioner), who are embarking on their first piece of research. The decisions that they have to make as they progress through their research projects are the same as the decisions you will have to make.

In a book of this size we obviously can't go into a huge amount of detail (particularly about methods of analysis, for example), but we aim to tell you what it is you need to know and do, and when you need to know and do it. We also suggest how to set about getting the help you need from a supervisor, a librarian, a statistician, other clinicians, colleagues, and so on.

We have aimed the book at the health research novice who may be working in any one of the many disciplines in health care, for example as a doctor, nurse, physiotherapist, health visitor, dietitian, occupational therapist, health promoter or health educator, to name a few.

We hope the book will also be of use to those who are acting as research supervisors for the first time (or who have a limited amount of supervision experience) – this book will provide you with a helpful framework of how a successful research project should be carried out.

The three authors have between them many years of experience of carrying out, teaching about, and supervising health research in a medical school attached to a major teaching hospital, and have themselves published a great many research papers.

David Bowers
Allan House
David Owens
University of Leeds, Institute of Health Sciences, 2011

I

Limbering Up

1

Turning Your General Aim Into a Specific Question

THE BEGINNING

Most people have a pretty good idea of the general area in which they want to research. A useful starting point is to ask yourself, 'What interests me about my own area and why?' You should keep this thought in mind as you plan your research – otherwise there is a real risk of getting drawn into doing something because it is feasible, or because somebody else wants you to, rather than because it answers your own questions.

WHAT ARE YOUR AIMS?

The next task is to start framing a *question* – to begin with in quite general terms. For example, suppose you are interested in the observation that not everybody goes to a doctor as soon as they have symptoms suggesting cancer. Your question might be: why is that? What are the personal, social and clinical factors that influence time to presentation of cancer? Or you might ask: does it matter? Do people who present quickly with symptoms do better than people who present late? And if so, why? Or you might decide you know enough about the answers to these questions, and you want to do something to reduce late presentations with cancer. So your question is: what could we do to reduce the time it takes for people to present symptoms to a doctor?

These general questions can be restated as the AIM or AIMS of a project. Aims are typically expressed as statements, such as this:

To determine whether a public education campaign reduces rates of late presentation with symptoms of bowel cancer.

Typically a study should have only *one* main or primary aim. It may have a couple of subsidiary or secondary aims. A good rule is that the smaller your study the fewer aims you should have. Most studies that have more than three or four aims do not achieve any of them.

WHAT IS YOUR QUESTION?

Once you have decided on your main aim, you need to frame one or more specific questions related to it. We will give an example a little later, but first a word about hypotheses.

Getting Started in Health Research, First Edition. David Bowers, Allan House and David Owens.
© 2011 David Bowers, Allan House and David Owens. Published 2011 by Blackwell Publishing Ltd.

Hypothesis is a Greek word that refers to a scientific proposition. For example, a hypothesis might be a theory put forward to explain a number of experimental observations. For our current purposes, we can think of it as a proposition about the likely findings of a piece of research. For example, we might hypothesize 'People who present late with symptoms suggestive of bowel cancer are less likely to have a relative who has had bowel cancer than are people who present early with symptoms.'

There used to be a vogue for expressing all hypotheses in the negative, the so-called 'null hypothesis', even when it was pretty obviously not what the investigator thought. Thus, 'People who present late with symptoms of cancer do no worse than people who present early.'

The reason for this convention is that certain statistical tests are designed to prove something *isn't* the case – typically that two groups of people or measurements have not come from the same population (for more on this you could do worse than look at Chapter 21 in *Understanding Clinical Papers* by we three authors (Bowers, House and Owens, 2006)). However, the null hypothesis convention does not make for easy reading and can lead to some pretty absurd-sounding propositions.

Not all hypotheses are tested by the use of statistics that refute a null hypothesis, and not all research questions are hypotheses. So the simplest way to proceed is always to think of your research as being designed to answer a simple and unambiguous question.

Sometimes researchers talk about aims and objectives rather than aims and hypotheses. This makes sense when what you are doing is just as well put as a statement. Here are some examples of research objectives:

- *To determine the prevalence of obesity among children entering secondary education at the age of 11 years.*
- *To determine the accuracy of prostate specific antigen (PSA) as a test for cancer among men seen in primary care, as part of a population-based screening programme.*

In the next section we want to introduce you to Dinesh and Anna, two (fictitious) characters, who are also about to start doing some research for the first time. We will use their research stories to illustrate, step by step, the tasks and challenges – and their solutions – which are commonly encountered by inexperienced (indeed by all) researchers.

GETTING THE QUESTION CLEAR

This is a two-stage process. Step 1 involves linking your aim to a *starter question*. Then Step 2 involves clarifying the meaning of every term in your starter question. As an example we can see how Dinesh and Anna got started with their research questions. We'll start with Dinesh.

Dinesh

Dinesh works as a nurse in the emergency department of a big inner-city hospital. He notices a problem with people who come to the department after they have harmed themselves, for example by cutting their arms or taking an overdose. Communication between these people and staff may be tense or difficult, and it is clear that both sides find the encounter unsatisfactory. One day he is talking to a friend who works in a health centre for asylum seekers where there is an advocacy service and the friend tells him how helpful it is.

Dinesh decides to plan a project. His *aim* is to establish the benefits of an advocacy service in his department. He decides his research question is as shown in Figure 1.1.

> Does providing an advocacy service lead to better outcomes for people who attend an emergency department after an act of self-harm?

FIGURE 1.1   Dinesh's first version of his 'starter' research question.

This seems a good start, but then he discusses his idea with another friend who is training to be an eye surgeon. This friend has no idea either what an advocacy service consists of or what constitutes good outcomes after an episode of self-harm. During their talk Dinesh scribbles some notes on his question (Figure 1.2).

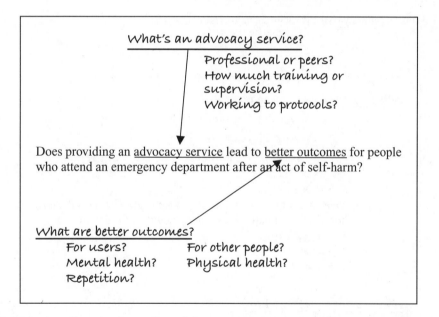

FIGURE 1.2   Dinesh realises that he needs to define some of the terms in his starter question – his proposed intervention and his desired outcome.

Next he goes to talk to his head of department, who asks some more questions. Who exactly might be offered this advocacy service? And at what stage in their journey through the department? So Dinesh does some more scribbling (Figure 1.3).

Dinesh's next step is a coffee with one of the more friendly psychiatrists who visits his department. The psychiatrist tells him that in his experience self-harm is quite diverse, so that Dinesh will need to decide what counts as an act of self-harm. And he also points out that delivering treatments can be a bit hit and miss, so that Dinesh needs to decide how much advocacy is enough to give it a fair trial. This is a bit like deciding what is a fair trial of physiotherapy after stroke. Dinesh has another go (Figure 1.4).

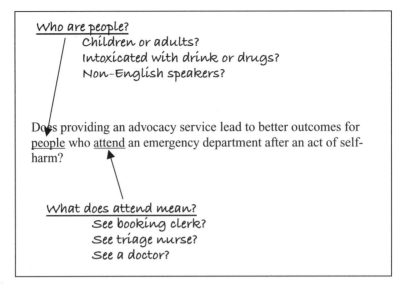

FIGURE 1.3   Dinesh defines who the participants in his research will be.

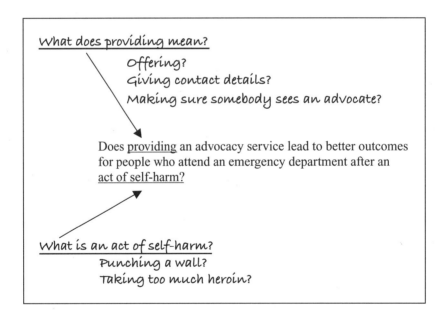

FIGURE 1.4   Dinesh looks at two terms in his question and tries to clarify what they mean.

Now Dinesh is in a position to state his question much more clearly and specifically – exactly what he means by advocacy, who it's for, how it's going to be delivered, and what outcomes he is interested in. This basic starter question may not change much, but Dinesh will spell out its meaning as he subsequently describes the methods of his study (see Chapter 6 onwards).

Anna

Anna is a general practitioner. She has a particular concern about the low take up of the MMR vaccine in her practice. In this she includes not only parents who won't bring their children at all, but also those who ask to have the components as individual jabs. She would like to find some way of improving the MMR take-up rate. She has tried writing to parents who have not brought their child for the jab, and has put posters up in the waiting area, and in all of the consulting rooms. She has also discussed the issue with those parents asking for separate jabs. But there has been no discernible increase in the MMR take-up rate. She realises that she needs to investigate further, and decides to carry out a research project. Anna's starter research question is shown in Figure 1.5.

> What would persuade reluctant parents to change their minds and bring their child to have the MMR jab?

FIGURE 1.5   Anna's first version of her 'starter' research question.

Anna thinks that she could use the patients in her own group practice to answer this question.

After discussing her project with colleagues in the practice and with a friend who works in public health, Anna realises that she does not know enough about why parents are reluctant – beyond being aware of a recent unfortunate scare campaign in the national press. She therefore modifies her question as shown in Figure 1.6.

> Why are parents reluctant to bring their children for MMR vaccination when advised by their GP that it's for the best?

FIGURE 1.6   Anna modifies her research question.

Anna decides she needs to think about this question further and she starts by thinking about the people involved (Figure 1.7).

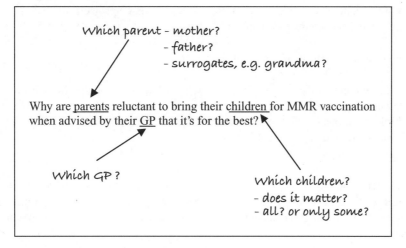

FIGURE 1.7   Anna notes that she needs to define some of the terms in her research question – exactly which people will be involved in her research?

Anna soon realises, however, that there are other components of her question that she needs to pick apart. She has another try (see Figure 1.8).

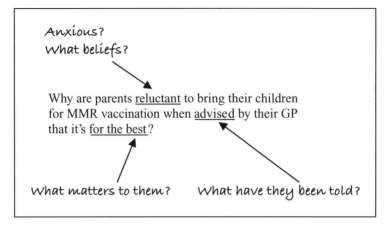

FIGURE 1.8   Anna also needs to define what she wants to learn from her study.

Anna now feels ready to state her question more clearly and to start thinking – about whom to interview and what questions to ask.

This approach to question setting will be familiar to anybody who has ever sat an essay exam because it is exactly same as the approach to question answering. It helps you make sure you have not forgotten anything and it's an extremely useful way of helping with planning the next stage – in our case, deciding on a design, subjects, measures, and so on. We will return to Dinesh and Anna in later chapters.

FINAL CHECKS

If you have followed this approach for your own project, you should by now have three statements:

- an outline of a general area of interest, with a statement about *why* it is interesting;
- a statement of the general aim or aims (caution!) of your research project;
- an unambiguous and specific research question.

The commonest mistakes people make at this stage are:

- making vague restatements of the area of interest – with the question couched in such terms as 'exploring issues' or 'identifying associations';
- posing multiple questions – either explicitly as a long list, or in a more covert way by posing a small number of compound or composite questions;
- using unclear terminology.

If you are confident that you have not made these mistakes – you are ready to move on. However, before you expend any more time and effort fruitlessly, you need to see if any other researcher has already tackled your proposed area of research. You can begin with a quick look at what's already been done – the subject of the next chapter.

2

Taking a Preliminary Look at What Has Already Been Done

IS THERE ANY POINT?

In the previous chapter we saw how both Dinesh and Anna sharpened up their research ideas, which enabled them to write down an unambiguous and specific research question. Basically, this is where we have got to:

- by now you know what the broad aim of your research is;
- you've got your research question sorted;
- you think that your project is going to be helpful to you professionally;
- it will be worthwhile, and will add to knowledge;
- it will be intellectually challenging;
- you believe that you will be able to see it through to the end.

However, you wonder what's the point of going any further if someone else has already done exactly what you plan to do? In fact you can repeat some previous research if you think it was in some way inadequate or flawed! Maybe there were methodological faults, or the results were misinterpreted, or unjustified; or the outcome was so startling that you feel that you would like to try and reproduce it. Or perhaps it was concerned with a quite different target population. Even a rather small sample size in a previous study might be a good enough reason to have another go yourself.

For example, here are the titles of a series of papers which all investigated the same thing: whether or not stress was a statistically significant risk factor for breast cancer in women:

Adverse life events and breast cancer: case-control study. Chen *et al.* (1995).

Stressful life events and difficulties and onset of breast cancer: case-control study. Protheroe *et al.* (1999).

Stressful life events and risk of breast cancer in 10 808 women: a cohort study. Lillberg *et al.* (2003).

Self-reported stress and risk of breast cancer: prospective cohort study. Nielsen *et al.* (2005).

Each successive author decided that they could, in some way, improve on the previous research.

Getting Started in Health Research, First Edition. David Bowers, Allan House and David Owens.
© 2011 David Bowers, Allan House and David Owens. Published 2011 by Blackwell Publishing Ltd.

In any case, you need to find out what's already out there before you go any further. How? In Chapter 4 we will examine this question in detail, but here we are going to have a quick glance over the barricade, to scope out the research landscape and see if anything noticeable is sticking up.

GATEWAYS – A SIMPLE WAY INTO SEARCHING

Here are a few things that you can do without (at this stage anyway) investing a huge amount of time.

➤ Use Google Scholar

As it says on the box, this 'provides a search of scholarly literature across many disciplines and sources, including theses, books, abstracts and articles.'

The web address is: http://google.scholar.co.uk[1]

But it is easier simply to type Google Scholar into Google, and select Google Scholar from the search results. Figure 2.1 shows the home page. You can now either type in one or more keywords into the Search box, or for a more refined search, click Advanced Google Scholar (as shown in Figure 2.2). If you click Advanced Search Tips you will be given advice on how to search more effectively, as well as getting access to Google Scholar help.

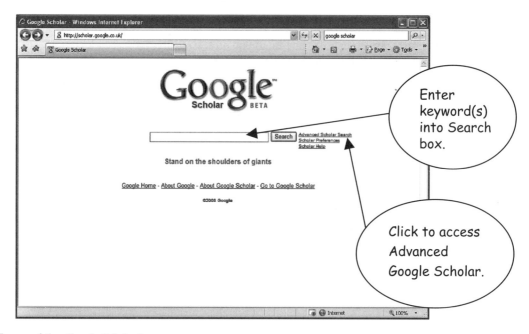

FIGURE 2.1   Google Scholar home page.

➤ Use PubMed®

This is a service of the US National Library of Medicine (NLM). The home page is shown in Figure 2.3.

The web address is: www.ncbi.nlm.nih.gov/pubmed/

---

[1]   Note: All web site addresses were last accessed in January 2011.

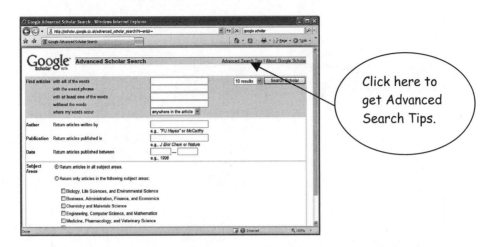

FIGURE 2.2   Advanced Google Scholar search page.

But perhaps the easiest way to access it is simply to type PubMed into Google and look for PubMed Home – it is usually at or near the top of the Google results page.

You can then type your key words into the Search box. If you want to find out how to use PubMed more effectively there is an excellent tutorial feature (see Figure 2.3).

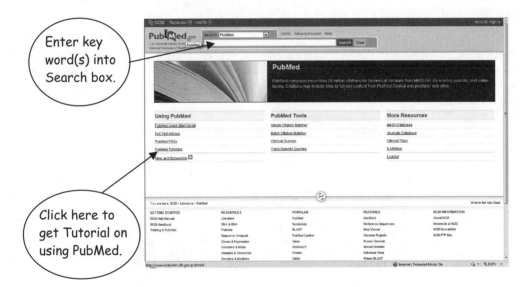

FIGURE 2.3   PubMed home page.

➤ Use CINAHL® (The Cumulative Index to Nursing and Allied Health Literature)

This database, as its title suggests, focuses on nursing and allied heath research. At the time of writing, it is no longer available for individual use, but most academic and clinical institutions will subscribe to it. The CINAHL home page is shown in Figure 2.4.

The web address is: www.cinahl.com

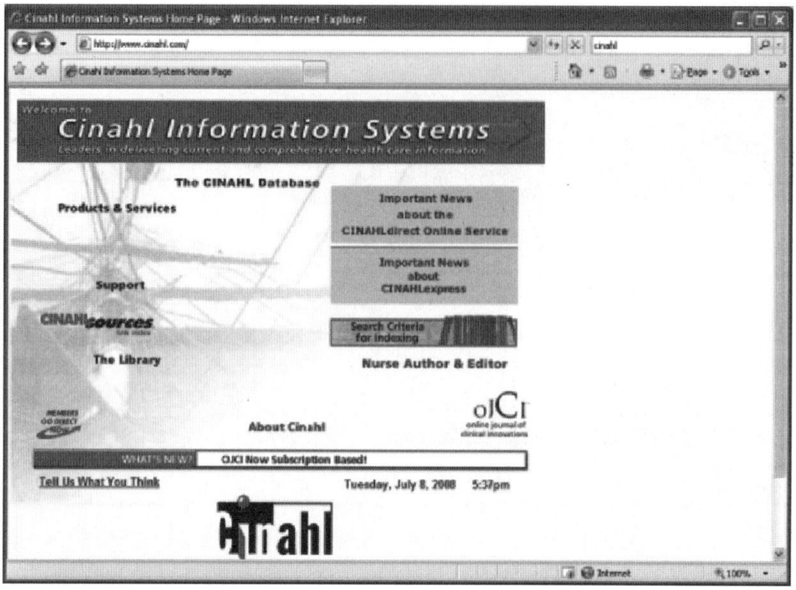

FIGURE 2.4 CINAHL homepage.

➤ Use the NLM (National Library of Medicine) Gateway®

The NLM Gateway describes itself as *'one-stop shopping'* for an increasing number of the information resources of the National Library of Medicine (NLM). It is targeted at the Internet user who comes to NLM not knowing exactly what is here, or how best to search for it. A single interface that searches in multiple retrieval systems, Gateway provides a single address, look, and feel. It currently accesses 21 databases, including PubMed.

The web address is: http://gateway.nlm.nih.gov

But once again, it is easier to type NLM Gateway into Google. The homepage is shown in Figure 2.5. You can enter your search keywords into the Search box as shown. More information, including a list

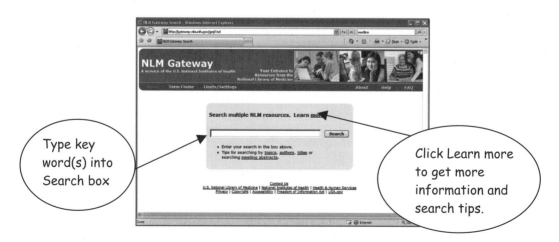

FIGURE 2.5 NLM Gateway homepage.

of the databases accessed by Gateway and some search tips, is available if you click 'Learn more' (see Figure 2.6).

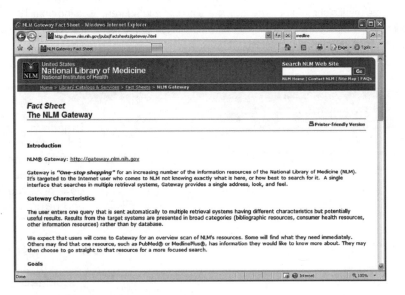

FIGURE 2.6   The first page of the NLM 'Learn more' page.

Searching PubMed, Google Scholar, NLM and CINAHL may well unearth previous work in your chosen area, but is not certain to do so. These databases can never be completely up to date, and they are not likely to include unpublished research. Moreover they may not include conference proceedings, unpublished theses, every non-English language research paper, pharmaceutical company reports, and so on. We will examine more comprehensive search procedures in Chapter 4 – this present chapter is after all only a guide to having a preliminary glance at the research territory – although there are a couple of other things you can do now.

YOU CAN TALK WITH COLLEAGUES

There are a couple of other things that you can do that will not involve a lot of effort and time. One of them is to talk to colleagues, or colleagues of colleagues. Or to people you know who are familiar with your chosen field, or to people those people may know. This sort of networking may sometimes yield pleasant (or unpleasant) surprises. Who knows – there may be relevant, ongoing, but as yet unpublished work out there which may be in your proposed research domain.

YOU CAN TALK TO YOUR ACADEMIC OR CLINICAL LIBRARIAN

It won't do any harm to visit and chat with your librarian, either academic or clinical. She or he will usually have their ear to the ground and may thus be able to tell you what's going on research-wise in and around their own institution. This will be particularly true if your library is big enough to have subject-specialist librarians. Besides, it's a good idea to make yourself known to the library people, even if they have nothing immediate to offer you. When you come to do the more intensive searches described in Chapter 4 you may be grateful for more specialist help.

Dinesh

For his preliminary search, Dinesh logs in to PubMed, and in the search box types: 'advocacy service for self-harm patients'. He gets the results shown in Figure 2.7. There is only one reference, dating from 1999, in the *BMJ*.

Dinesh knows that he must read this material, but is comforted by the fact that there doesn't seem to be much else already out there. It seems OK to proceed – for the moment anyway.

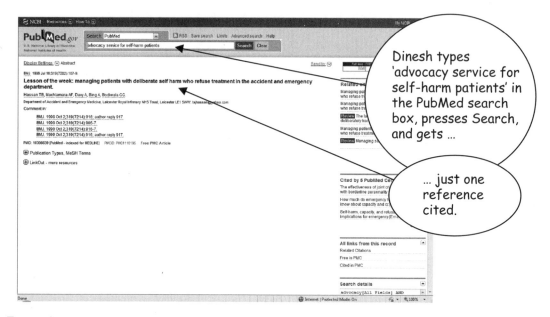

FIGURE 2.7   The PubMed results after Dinesh typed in 'advocacy service for self-harm patients'.

When it comes to making a more thorough and systematic search (see Chapter 4) a helpful guide will be the acronym *PICOS*, standing for: **P**atient population (and disease of interest); **I**ntervention; **C**omparator; **O**utcome; and **S**tudy design (type of) to be included. In anticipation of his systematic search Dinesh jots down his PICOS parameters as shown in Figure 2.8.

> Population: Self-harm patients attending an ED.
> Intervention: Use of an advocacy service.
> Comparator: Similar patients not using an advocacy service.
> Outcome: Re-attendance time. Mood. Satisfaction.
> Study design: Clinical trial (possibly – but not decided yet –
>   see Chapter 6).

FIGURE 2.8   Dinesh's PICOS parameters.

He is then able to re-phrase his research question (first noted in Chapter 1) as shown in Figure 2.9. Notice that he interprets 'better outcomes' as longer time to re-attendance and improved mood.

Do patients attending an ED after an
episode of self-harm who use an
advocacy service have a longer time to
re-attendance and improved mood
compared to similar patients who do not
use an advocacy service, as measured
by a clinical trial?

FIGURE 2.9   Dinesh modifies his research question by defining what he means by 'better outcomes'.

He knows that it will pay to make contact with colleagues, and with authors publishing in the same field wherever he can find them, so as to locate ongoing but unpublished studies. Librarians (information experts) can be immensely helpful, so he'll fix a meeting with his librarian. His objective is to identify studies with the same PICOS profile as his own.

Dinesh will need to describe all of this in his search protocol: which databases, which other resources, which search terms to be used with electronic databases, and so on. He decides on several database search terms, some of which are shown in Figure 2.10. He will return to this list when he visits his local librarian and we will discuss it further in Chapter 4.

(self-harm OR suicide) AND clinical trial
Patient advocate AND clinical trial
Patient advocacy service
Patient advocacy service AND clinical trial
(self-harm OR suicide) re-attendance
(self-harm OR suicide) repetition
(self-harm OR suicide) AND emergency department

FIGURE 2.10   Dinesh has a go at writing down some possible database search terms.

Anna

Anna talks to everyone she thinks might know of work having been done (or currently being done) in her subject area. However, she doesn't get any particularly helpful responses. She decides to have a look on the Internet, and although appropriate search terms for her qualitative research may perhaps be a little less cut and dried than Dinesh's, she can still have a look at what's out there. She thinks that she will need to search for any MMR references around keywords like 'attitudes', 'beliefs', and so on. She makes the following note of some potentially relevant search terms (see Figure 2.11).

Anna decides that rather than using PubMed and Google Scholar, a better place for her to start might be PsycINFO®, the search facility on the website of the American Psychological Association, at www.apa.org/psycinfo (once again it's easier to type psycinfo into Google or Bing, etc.).

MMR OR vaccination AND attitudes or beliefs

Parents OR mother OR carer OR patient

FIGURE 2.11   Anna's database search terms.

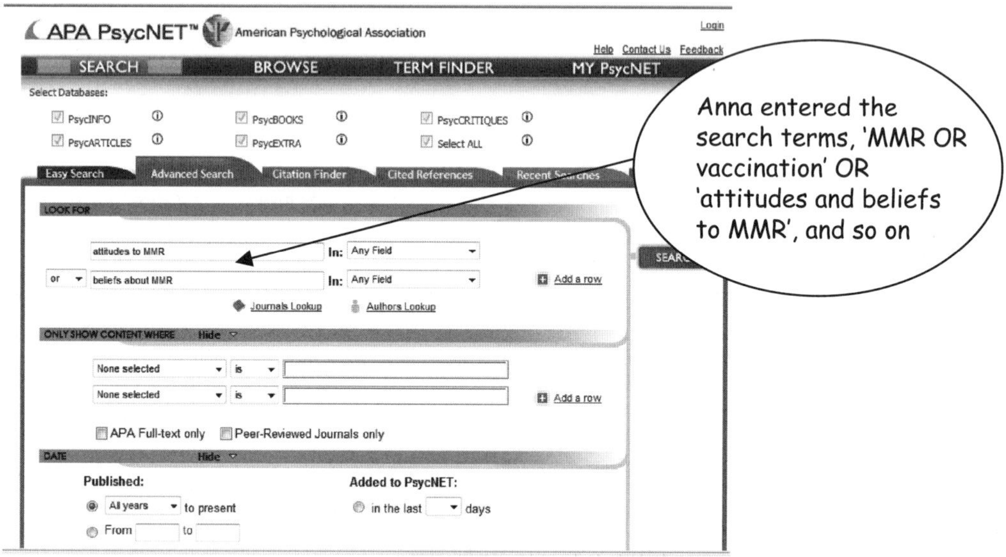

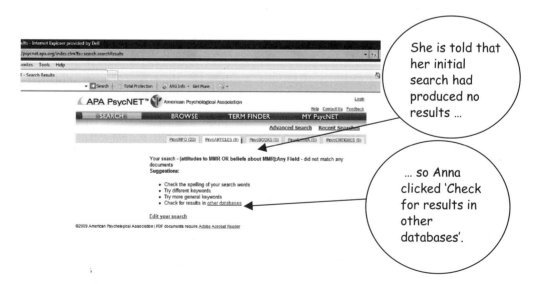

FIGURE 2.12   Anna has typed her search terms into the PsycINFO search boxes.

FIGURE 2.13   Anna is told that there are no hits with the PsycINFO databases, and clicks the 'Check for results in other databases' field.

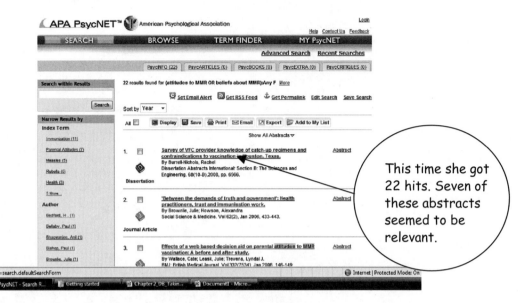

FIGURE 2.14   Anna gets 22 hits from the other databases searched.

In the PsycINFO search box she types in the search terms shown in Figure 2.11 (see Figure 2.12), but gets no hits (Figure 2.13), so clicks <Check for results in other databases>, and gets 22 hits (Figure 2.14). She reads the abstracts and finds that seven of these articles may be relevant.

Anna reads all of these references carefully, but decides that either they do not match her own research intentions, or they are in some other way unsuitable (too small a sample, different population, and so on). She feels confident that she can at least proceed to the next stage.

Let's assume that by using some or all of the above resources, you have satisfied yourself that all is well, that no one else has covered the same ground, and you feel happy and ready to proceed. You have made a note of the more detailed search strategy you are likely to need in due course, and you keep it to discuss with your local librarian. But first you now need to prepare a preliminary *research protocol* – which is (in brief) a concise written plan of the work you intend to do, outlining each step of the process. We will see how this is done in the next chapter.

On Your Marks

3

Coming Up With an Initial Plan of Action

THE INITIAL PLAN

Suppose you now have a fairly good idea about your question, and you have quickly checked the literature for what has been done before. The next step is to start sketching out the sort of study you might undertake to answer your question. What you should do is draft out the first part of an action plan – outlining something about these design aspects of your study. Later (see Chapter 14) you will refine this and add some sections on implementation of your research.

A typical (brief) research protocol might have the headings shown in Figure 3.1.

- background
- aims and hypotheses (objectives)
- methods
  - design
  - setting
  - sample
  - measures
  - data analysis
- feasibility
- ethical considerations
- support

FIGURE 3.1   A simple format for a research protocol.

STUDY DESIGN

You would start therefore with notes about a study design. Let's see what Dinesh and Anna might do.

Dinesh

For example – Dinesh knows that he wants to understand the impact of a new service offered in the emergency department. He makes a note of some candidate designs (see Figure 3.2) and moves on – he will discuss which one to choose with his research mentor.

Getting Started in Health Research, First Edition. David Bowers, Allan House and David Owens.
© 2011 David Bowers, Allan House and David Owens. Published 2011 by Blackwell Publishing Ltd.

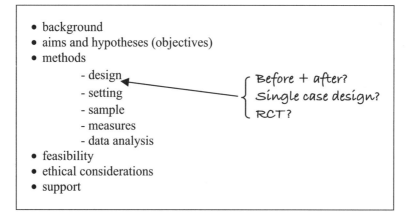

• background
• aims and hypotheses (objectives)
• methods
    - design
    - setting
    - sample
    - measures
    - data analysis
• feasibility
• ethical considerations
• support

Before + after?
Single case design?
RCT?

FIGURE 3.2   Dinesh starts to use his protocol headings to think about some possible research designs.

Anna

Anna also thinks about study design. She realises pretty quickly that she wants to study peoples' attitudes on (for now anyway) a single occasion. She decides that a questionnaire will be too rigid – she wants to be able to explore in a fairly free way what people think – and decides to opt for an interview with parents. She is not sure yet whether this is really research but it does seem the best way to get at reasons for reluctance to take up the MMR vaccine.

We will discuss designs in detail (as you will do with your mentor) in Chapter 6. For now, you can proceed with the next part of your protocol – deciding *where* you are going to do your research.

CHOOSING A SETTING

Most of us do not have much choice about where we do our first research study. You are probably working, for example, in a place that means you have access to just one or two clinics (if it is patients you want to research), or one or two wards or primary care surgeries. That may not be a problem, but be cautious – sometimes working in specialist settings can lead to unexpected biases.

(1)   Specialist centres recruit difficult cases (see Figure 3.3).
      In this review the authors showed that the answer to the question, 'How frequently does a baby who has had a febrile seizure go on to have a non-febrile seizure?', depends where you are when you ask the question! The obvious explanation is that clinics in secondary and tertiary care see more complicated cases – seriously ill children or those with multiple other problems.
(2)   Taking a sample from one clinic at one time leads to chronic cases being over-represented (see Figure 3.4).
      This figure shows the duration of illness of nine people, three of whom are chronic cases – their illness lasts longer than one of the epochs marked by the vertical lines. However, if you collected cases at one point in time (marked by the dotted vertical line) in one clinic, you would conclude that three-quarters of the cases of the condition ran a chronic course.

Sample Selection and the Natural History of Disease. Studies of Febrile Seizures.

Ellenberg JH, Nelson KB

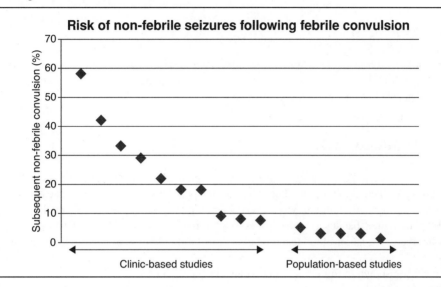

FIGURE 3.3   Specialist centres recruit complex cases. An example taken from a study of non-febrile seizures following febrile convulsions.

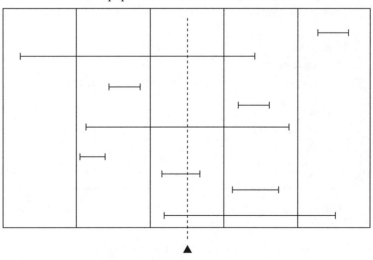

FIGURE 3.4   Sampling in one clinic at one time can lead to chronic cases being over-represented.

Dinesh

For now, Dinesh decides that – since his emergency department is the only one in a reasonably typical city – the first problem does not apply. And since his department sees all-comers, and does not book follow-ups, then he won't be seeing chronic cases (although he may well see repeat attenders).

DECIDING ON A SAMPLE

We discuss the logic of choosing a sample (those subjects who will participate in your research), and how to do it, in Chapters 7 and 8. At this stage you just need to think about the reasons why you would choose the sample, so you can discuss them with your mentor.

DECIDING ON MEASURES

Some measures are designed to put a study in context for the reader. For example, measures that describe the volume and type of activity in a particular service or the population served by it: these can help a reader decide how like their own environment was the one in which the research was conducted.

   Then there are measures that describe the processes you are studying. For example, if it's an investigation study then what types of scan or blood test are being done? Finally you will need to think about measures of outcomes.

   Dinesh's notes are shown in Figure 3.5, and Anna's in Figure 3.6.

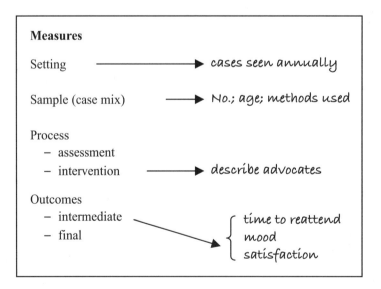

FIGURE 3.5   Dinesh makes an initial note of the things he might want to measure in his research.

   With your protocol this well developed, you are now in a position to share your ideas with your mentor or supervisor. You have a clear idea of your question and what work has gone before, and some preliminary ideas about how to research your topic. Do not do more at this stage! Your mentor is likely to discuss changes, and it can be frustrating for both of you if you have done too much detailed planning at this stage and then have to change it all!

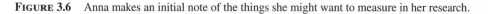

Measures

Setting: *Our practice*
                                - list size
                                - no. of babies
                                - current take -up rate

Sample: *Start with mums for first study*

Process:
  - assessment   *Note length of interview*
  - intervention   *Need a topic guide for the interview*

Outcomes   *What will these look like in my study?*

FIGURE 3.6   Anna makes an initial note of the things she might want to measure in her research.

So far, so good. Now you need to do a really thorough search of the literature. Although you didn't turn anything up with your quick search (Chapter 2), you now need to make absolutely sure that nobody else has properly answered your research question. We'll see how you can do this in the next chapter.

4

Carrying Out a Systematic Search

HAVING A MUCH CLOSER LOOK

In Chapter 2 you had a quick look (principally using Google Scholar and PubMed) for any evidence of previous work by other researchers in your proposed research area, and found nothing to prevent you carrying on. But before you go any further you've absolutely got to go beyond this cursory look and do a much more thorough and systematic search to make completely sure – it would be a pity to get several months in and then stumble across a paper that had already pretty much answered your own research question.

You may have heard of a systematic review, the objective of which is to summarise the totality of evidence on a specific clinical subject in an organised way and following a set protocol. We should note right now that for some people the term 'systematic review' is synonymous with a review process that is concluded with a meta-analysis. For them, a systematic review is incomplete without this synthesising final step. However, this is not necessary here. Dinesh is only interested in what relevant research may have already been carried out. He's not interested in any form of data synthesis, although of course some research projects may well take the form of a meta-analysis.

Even though you don't want to do a systematic review complete with its meta-analysis, you can still use the same sort of systematic protocol-guided approach (which we will illustrate below), and you should write this protocol before you start your search. By the way, you will obviously need to check that there hasn't already been a systematic review in your own topic. You can do this with:

- the Cochrane Library (www.cochranelibrary.com)
- the NHS Centre for Reviews and Dissemination (www.york.ac.uk/inst/crd/welcome.htm)
- and PubMed, using the appropriate search filters.

The design and implementation of a systematic review is an extensive and fairly demanding subject area (remember, you are only doing the searching bit). We can't do more than give the barest outlines here, but the following couple of sources offer a comprehensive and detailed account of the process:

- http://www.york.ac.uk/inst/crd/report4.htm
- http://www.medicine.ox.ac.uk/bandolier/painres/download/whatis/Health-util.pdf

Getting Started in Health Research, First Edition. David Bowers, Allan House and David Owens.
© 2011 David Bowers, Allan House and David Owens. Published 2011 by Blackwell Publishing Ltd.

THE SYSTEMATIC REVIEW PROTOCOL

The six elements of the systematic review protocol are as follows:

(1) *The formulation of a focussed review question*, with clearly defined inclusion (and exclusion) criteria. You will recall that Dinesh's PICOS parameters (see Chapter 2, p. 14) led him to the research question shown in Figure 4.1.

> Do patients attending an ED after an episode of self-harm who use an advocacy service have a longer time to re-attendance and improved mood compared to similar patients who do not use an advocacy service, as measured by a clinical trial?

FIGURE 4.1   Dinesh's research question again (see Figure 2.9).

(2) *A description of your search strategy.*
      You will need to make an exhaustive search of published and unpublished reports, including non-English sources (to avoid language bias). The sources you will need to search include those shown in Figure 4.2.

> Appropriate databases (see Chapter 2)
>
> Other appropriate internet sources (search engines)
>
> Journal articles and other research papers (including references)
>
> Conference proceedings (and any references)
>
> Pharmaceutical, and other relevant company, reports
>
> Theses, dissertations, textbooks, citations, and so on
>
> Colleagues, acknowledged experts, librarians

FIGURE 4.2   Some common sources of research articles.

We should note, to be honest, that it's very difficult to locate unpublished studies, particularly those not in English. Systematic reviews are therefore nearly always likely to be incomplete. All you can do is keep your fingers crossed.

You will recall that in Chapter 2 we outlined the process needed to do a preliminary search, and then, in a little more detail, had a look at what Dinesh and Anna decided.

An example of a database search strategy is shown in Figure 4.3, an extract from a study into the cardiovascular effects of marine omega-3 fatty acids.

But when it comes to a fully detailed systematic search you will rarely see one described in the literature, and at this point you really do need to consult an information specialist – one is probably to be found in your nearest academic library. The Cochrane Library database (www.cochrane.org)

Cardiovascular effects of marine omega-3 fatty acids

Palaniappan Saravanan, Neil Davidson, Erik B Schmidt, Philip C Calder

Search strategy and selection criteria: We searched Medline, Embase, the Cochrane Library, PubMed, CINAHL, IPA, Web of Science, Scopus, and Pascal for reports published between January 1970 and January 2010. We used the search terms 'omega-3 fatty acids' or 'n-3 PUFA' in combination with the terms 'cardiac', 'cardio-vascular', 'sudden cardiac death', 'arrhythmia', 'ion channels', 'atrial fibrillation', 'stroke', 'hypertension', 'triglycerides', 'immunology', and 'inflammation'. We largely selected publications from the past 15 years, but did not exclude commonly referenced and highly regarded older publications. We also searched the reference lists of articles identified by this search strategy and selected those we judged relevant.

FIGURE 4.3   An example of a database search strategy from a study into the cardiovascular effects of marine omega-3 fatty acids.

provides a complete and detailed description of thousands of systematic searches. Figure 4.4 is the abstract and a description of one such search; this related to the treatment of fetal lung maturation.

You will find it helpful to store all of your identified studies in some appropriate reference database, for example EndNote (www.endnote.com), or Reference Manager (www.refman.com). This will enable you to manage what eventually might be a large number of references. The software chosen for this task should be noted in your protocol. This resource will also be helpful when you come to write up your research findings (see Chapters 21 and 22).

(3) *Study selection.*

Inevitably, not all of the studies you locate will be entirely appropriate for one reason or another, so now you have to start weeding out those which don't quite fit the bill. It is important that you avoid selection bias when you do this, and your protocol should specify the process by which studies will be selected, principally your *inclusion and exclusion criteria*. These criteria will necessarily follow from your defined PICOS parameters. Ideally there should be two of you involved in the selection process (to reduce subjectivity). How you will resolve any differences between you in selection decisions (by arbitration, for example) should also be described.

As an example, Figure 4.5 describes the study selection process undertaken by the authors of a systematic review of cohort studies of the association of bodyweight with total mortality and cardiovascular events in coronary artery disease.

(4) *Study quality assessment.*

Even if you find a study (or studies) that appears to cover the research you propose, this doesn't mean that you must necessarily abandon your own work. It may be that the quality of the study is poor, and you feel therefore that the conclusions reached are likely to be unreliable. Or perhaps the conclusions don't match the results. Or the sample is small. This means that you need to examine the *quality* of your selected studies – mainly their internal validity (lack of bias) – using pre-determined quality criteria which must be described in your protocol. These will vary according to the study design.

For example, if you are searching randomised controlled trials, issues like randomisation and blinding will be important quality criteria; if case-control studies, the number of controls and the method of their selection can be assessed. The number of quality reviewers (again a minimum of two of you working independently, with a stated means of resolving disagreements) must also be specified in your protocol. The end result of this process will be a final set of studies which may be arranged in some sort of quality hierarchy. As an example, Figure 4.6 is from the same paper as that in the previous section. As you can see, the judging of quality can be complex!

Antenatal corticosteroids for accelerating fetal lung maturation for women at risk of preterm birth

Roberts D, Dalziel S

Cochrane Database of Systematic Reviews 2006 Issue 3. Copyright © 2006 The Cochrane Collaboration. Published by John Wiley & Sons, Ltd.

Abstract

Background: Respiratory distress syndrome (RDS) is a serious complication of preterm birth and the primary cause of early neonatal mortality and disability.

Objectives: To assess the effects on fetal and neonatal morbidity and mortality, on maternal mortality and morbidity, and on the child in later life of administering corticosteroids to the mother before anticipated preterm birth.

Search strategy: We searched the Cochrane Pregnancy and Childbirth Group Trials Register (30 October 2005).

Selection criteria: Randomised controlled comparisons of antenatal corticosteroid administration (betamethasone, dexamethasone, or hydrocortisone) with placebo or with no treatment given to women with a singleton or multiple pregnancy, expected to deliver preterm as a result of either spontaneous preterm labour, preterm prelabour rupture of the membranes or elective preterm delivery.

Data collection and analysis: Two review authors assessed trial quality and extracted data independently.

Description of studies:
See table: Characteristics of Included Studies

Twenty-one studies met our inclusion criteria, with data available for 3885 women and 4269 infants. Six new studies have been included since the previous review involving 802 women and 819 infants (Amorim, 1999; Dexiprom, 1999; Fekih, 2002; Lewis, 1996; Nelson, 1985; Qublan, 2001).

Six of the included studies used dexamethasone as the corticosteroid in the treatment arm (1391 women and 1514 infants), while 14 studies used betamethasone (2476 women and 2737 infants) and one study did not specify the corticosteroid used (Cararach, 1991; 18 women and infants).

The included studies were conducted over a wide range of gestational ages, including those of extreme prematurity; obstetric indications for recruitment were premature rupture of membranes, spontaneous preterm labour and planned preterm delivery.

The included studies came from a range of healthcare systems and treatment eras. Ten of the studies were conducted in the USA, with two studies conducted in Finland and one study from each of the following countries; Brazil, Spain, South Africa, Canada, Tunisia, UK, New Zealand, Jordan, and The Netherlands. Six of the included studies completed recruitment mainly in the 1970s (1753 women and 1994 infants), six of the included studies completed recruitment mainly in the 1980s (1100 women and 1173 infants), and nine of the included studies completed recruitment mainly in the 1990s (1032 women and 1102 infants).

FIGURE 4.4 An abstract and description of a systematic search into the use of antenatal corticosteroids for fetal lung maturation. Taken from the Cochrane Library database.

Association of bodyweight with total mortality and with cardiovascular events in coronary artery disease: a systematic review of cohort studies

Abel Romero-Corral, Victor M Montori, Prof Virend K Somers, Josef Korinek, Randal J Thomas, Thomas G Allison, Farouk Mookadam, Francisco Lopez-Jimenez

Two investigators independently assessed the studies for eligibility. Inclusion criteria were: (1) studies including patients with CAD (defined as a history of percutaneous coronary intervention (PCI)), coronary artery bypass graft (CABG), or myocardial infarction (MI), at baseline – we did not include studies defining CAD with non-invasive techniques alone, such as treadmill test, coronary calcium score using CT, self-reported artery disease, or angina; (2) cohort studies with six months or longer of follow-up (studies with only in-hospital mortality data were not included); (3) reported risk estimates or number of events for total mortality, cardiovascular mortality, infarction, reinfarction, revacularisation, and major adverse events based on measures of bodyweight, such as BMI, percentage of excess weight, percentage body fat, waist circumference, or waist to hip ratio.

FIGURE 4.5   An example of a study selection process illustrating the types of studies which the authors included in their systematic review (from a study of bodyweight with mortality and cardiovascular events).

Association of bodyweight with total mortality and with cardiovascular events in coronary artery disease: a systematic review of cohort studies

Abel Romero-Corral, Victor M Montori, Prof Virend K Somers, Josef Korinek, Randal J Thomas, Thomas G Allison, Farouk Mookadam, Francisco Lopez-Jimenez

Quality assessment

Two reviewers independently assessed the quality of the manuscripts using the approaches recommended by Khan and colleagues and Stroup and colleagues for cohort studies. The main criterion were: (1) description of cardiovascular risk factors for each bodyweight group at baseline; (2) stage of CAD at enrolment (e.g. similar rates of previous PCI, CABG or MI, similar number of vessels diseased, similar angiographic characteristics); (3) history of PCI, CABG, or MI reliably ascertained (preferably with description of the technique used or the criteria used to assess MI, or both); (4) similarity of weight groups regarding cardiovascular risk factors such as age, sex, smoking, hypertension, etc.; (5) adjustment for the effect of these confounding variables (good adjustment judges to be controlling for age, sex and cardiovascular risk factors, adequate adjustment controlling for age and sex, and poor adjustment judged to be no intention to have controlled for known confounding factors); (6) those assessing outcome unaware of bodyweight; and (7) percentage of the cohort analysed at follow-up – quality was assigned as A or excellent with 6–8 points, B or good with 4–5, and C or sub-optimal with 0–3 points.

FIGURE 4.6   An example of quality assessment showing the quality criteria selected by the authors of the bodyweight and mortality with cardiovascular events study.

(5) *Data extraction.*

Your *protocol* should set out what information will be extracted from your selected studies. This will usually comprise study methodology, population, intervention(s), and outcome(s). Accuracy and consistency is vital in data extraction and because the process is prone to human error, it is best done with a *data extraction form*, which should contain clear instructions about coding the data.

If you envisage having to collect and store large amounts of data, you might want to consider an electronic data entry form which can be designed with, for example, Microsoft *Access*, or the more sophisticated *Visual FoxPro* (http://msdn.microsoft.com/en-gb/vfoxpro/bb190288.aspx), or more simply in a spreadsheet such as Microsoft *Excel*.

The design of your data extraction form and the number of independent reviewers (at least two, with a stated means of resolving discrepancies) must be detailed in your protocol, along with a note of the software package in which your data will be stored.

An example of data extraction methods is given in Figure 4.7, which is from a paper on radiotherapy methods for the treatment of head and neck cancer.

Hyperfractionated or accelerated radiotherapy in head and neck cancer: a meta-analysis

Prof Jean Bourhis, Prof Jens Overgaard, Héléne Audry, Prof Kian K Ang, Prof Michele Saunders, Jacques Bernier, Prof Jean-Claude Horiot, Aurélie Le Maître, Thomas F Pajak, Michael G Poulsen, Prof Brian O'Sullivan, Werner Dobrowsky, Prof Andrzej Hliniak, Krzysztof Skladowski, John H Hay, Luiz HJ Pinto, Carlo Fallai, Karen K Fu, Richard Sylvester, Dr Jean-Pierre Pignon, on behalf of the Meta-Analysis of Radiotherapy in Carcinomas of Head and neck (MARCH) Collaborative Group

---

Data extraction

The data requested for all patients were age, sex, tumour site, T and N classification, stage, histology, performance status, allocated treatment, and date of randomisation. The date and types of the first tumour failure, local, regional, or distant, and the date of secondary primary cancer were also recorded. Updated survival status and date of last follow-up were requested from the trialists. Data for patients excluded from the analysis after randomisation were obtained wherever possible.

FIGURE 4.7   A data extraction example, showing the variables on which the authors collected data (from a study of radiotherapy in head and neck cancer).

---

(6) *Data synthesis.*

Note again that if you are simply searching to reassure yourself that your research has not been done before, then you probably won't be interested in the data synthesis aspect of systematic review, and you will thus not need to read the rest of this section. You can present the results of your search in summary form with a commentary but no statistical analysis – sometimes called a narrative review.

The aim of data synthesis is to collect and summarise the results from the studies included in your review.

Principally, however, these results will be effect measures (differences in means or proportions, odds or risk ratios, sensitivities/specificities, p-values, and so on). An important aspect of the summary is that it provides evidence of the degree of consistency of the effects. Effects which vary noticeably from study to study are said to be heterogeneous. If your results are heterogeneous (and heterogeneity can be tested for with statistical computer programs) you will need to try and find an explanation for the condition.

Your summary may be descriptive, that is, non-quantitative, with a tabulated and/or graphical summary of the results (commonly, a *forest plot*). Alternatively, provided that your results are reasonably homogeneous, you may undertake a quantitative summary, that is, a pooling of results using a procedure such as a meta-analysis. Your protocol will need to specify what method of synthesis you intend, as well as the effect measure you are using.

A pooled effect is essentially a weighted average of all the studies, where the weights are commonly in proportion to sample size (or sometimes quality). Studies with large sample sizes are given more prominence. Software is available for meta-analysis. For example, Review Manager (RevMan) is available free from http://ims.cochrane.org/revman; or Stata, which can be bought from www.stata.com.

Finally, if you have conducted a meta-analysis you should test for publication bias. This can arise because statistically significant studies are more likely to be both submitted and accepted for publication. You can test for this using a *funnel plot*.

QUALITATIVE SYSTEMATIC REVIEWS

Although it is possible to conduct a systematic search for relevant qualitative studies (see, for example, Campbell *et al.* (2003))[1], the traditional systematic review framework is not well suited to qualitative research. For example, the search process itself may be more difficult because of research outcomes which are more subjective in nature than those for quantitative research. This means that it can be difficult to define appropriate search terms for electronic searching. Data synthesis (if carried out) is more likely to be descriptive (or in narrative form) and the problems associated with meta-analyses of qualitative effects have not been entirely resolved.

Anna

You will recall that Anna discovered a number of possibly relevant articles with her preliminary search (see Chapter 2). She decided to use a narrative summary of these results and any others that she might discover from a further, more organised search of the literature. She undertook a thematic analysis of the papers she found. To do this she first identified all the reasons given in the literature on why parents decline MMR. She then organised them into a small number of themes or categories. As she read more she had to modify her categories – adding a new one, broadening another, and changing its name. Eventually she ended up with five themes that seemed to her to describe all of the answers she got. Finally she enlisted help from a colleague to review the themes and the responses she had put in each one. As a result of discussions with the colleague she made some minor changes – moving a couple of items and changing the name of a theme – and was then able to write her summary of the qualitative literature.

---

[1] We are not in general providing references unless we feel that they are particularly important. See also Joannabriggs.edu.au/ CQRMG.

CONCLUSION

If your systematic search shows no significant evidence of previous work in your proposed research topic, then hallelujah, you can proceed with your research, comforted by the knowledge that you are (probably) the first there! And this is about the time when you should think about who might be able to help you in your project.

5

Building a Team

THE NEED FOR OTHER PEOPLE

The tasks set out so far (in Chapters 1 to 4) could be undertaken by a researcher on his or her own, perhaps with some judicious one-off help from specialists such as the librarian. But successful research, even in the case of small projects, is a highly collaborative activity. From this point onwards you need to recruit others who will help you take the ideas forward. So who needs to be on your team?

You may have read many research reports in the journals, and perhaps perused several dissertations or theses. These accounts of the research often don't do justice to the collaboration and assistance that has taken place. Only rarely are the roles of the people involved set out in any detail, although some journals sensibly insist on a brief tally of who did what.

Figure 5.1 is an example of the good publishing practice in which each author's contribution must be set out for the reader to see; this procedure helps to prevent people (often senior ones) who have done little or nothing from being included as authors (see the section on Authorship, Chapter 23). What is plain in this example is that there are lots of tasks in bringing a piece of research through to completion.

First, notice that four of the six authors were involved at an early stage: coming up with the research question, planning how to answer it, and applying for permission to carry it out. Three of the six were supervisors of the first author – who was undertaking the work for an MSc dissertation. She was assisted in the field work (in this case extracting data from a database) by another author, and two of her other colleagues helped with the management of the research data captured by the study. The first author was then assisted by two others in the analysis but drafted the manuscript alone – although all the authors helped to bring it to its final form.

In the next example (Figure 5.2) much the same kind of authorship statement provides a similar story, but this time many more people are thanked – most of them not authors of the paper. Five of the first author's colleagues are thanked specifically for their field work and data collection; many more are acknowledged rather generally for advice and support.

The team that a researcher builds up to deliver a finished project often emerges gradually. Members of the team will come and go at different stages and it will not necessarily be clear at the outset who will have the larger and smaller tasks, who will make the most effort, and who will have input at multiple stages of the research. Decisions about who might be authors of one or more paper at the end cannot usually be settled at the start of the project; the code for authorship (see Chapter 23) demands that substantial contributions have been made and usually that there is more intellectual input than data collection alone. Best not to promise authorship in haste and face the awkward job of backtracking from it later when the person's contribution doesn't reach the necessary level.

Getting Started in Health Research, First Edition. David Bowers, Allan House and David Owens.
© 2011 David Bowers, Allan House and David Owens. Published 2011 by Blackwell Publishing Ltd.

Bullous pemphigoid and pemphigus vulgaris—incidence and mortality in the UK: population based cohort study

S M Langan, research fellow,[1] L Smeeth, professor of clinical epidemiology,[2] R Hubbard, professor of respiratory epidemiology,[3] K M Fleming, research associate,[3] C J P Smith, senior research fellow,[3] J West, clinician scientist[3]

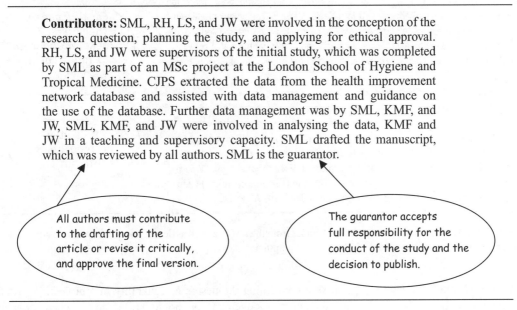

Contributors: SML, RH, LS, and JW were involved in the conception of the research question, planning the study, and applying for ethical approval. RH, LS, and JW were supervisors of the initial study, which was completed by SML as part of an MSc project at the London School of Hygiene and Tropical Medicine. CJPS extracted the data from the health improvement network database and assisted with data management and guidance on the use of the database. Further data management was by SML, KMF, and JW, SML, KMF, and JW were involved in analysing the data, KMF and JW in a teaching and supervisory capacity. SML drafted the manuscript, which was reviewed by all authors. SML is the guarantor.

All authors must contribute to the drafting of the article or revise it critically, and approve the final version.

The guarantor accepts full responsibility for the conduct of the study and the decision to publish.

FIGURE 5.1   Extract from a research paper from the *BMJ*, a journal that insists on details about each author's contribution.

WHO IS TO BE ON THE TEAM?

A supervisor

Where possible, a supervisor is likely to be the most valuable recruit for a researcher who is inexperienced. It isn't always possible to find the right person; we have substantial personal experience of unsupervised research in earlier years. It is an uphill struggle, too often accompanied by errors of judgement that could have been averted by advice from a reasonably wise supervisor. On the other hand a poor supervisor can, of course, be disastrous. How are you to select? There isn't usually an array of attractive candidates and, as in so many other areas, the few best people may be severely overloaded and either turn you down or agree but be less helpful than you hoped, because of their unavailability.

We have found it important to be wary of two kinds of supervisors. First, there is your senior colleague. Perhaps he or she (let's say he) is your manager or your boss in some way and is encouraging you to research, perhaps offering ideas from his own interests or your shared area of work. But as well as an enthusiasm for the topic, if he is to supervise, he needs to know about the process of research – so he should have substantial research experience as well as the clinical and seniority credentials. He should also be currently active in research; be very careful if he isn't.

Second, there are very senior researchers, awash with funding, holding unfeasibly large grants, and perhaps stars of the international conference circuit. There is a risk to you, the new researcher, that they may give you too little of their time. In addition, though, some of these experienced people have

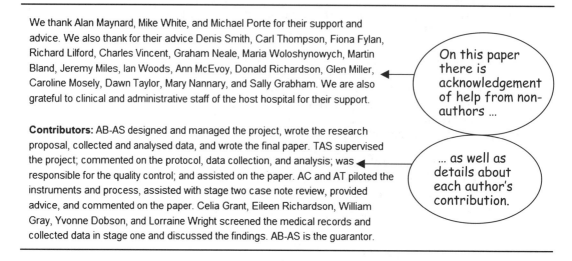

Sensitivity of routine system for reporting patient safety incidents in an NHS hospital: retrospective patient case note review

Ali Baba-Akbari Sari, Trevor A Sheldon, Alison Cracknell, Alastair Turnbull

We thank Alan Maynard, Mike White, and Michael Porte for their support and advice. We also thank for their advice Denis Smith, Carl Thompson, Fiona Fylan, Richard Lilford, Charles Vincent, Graham Neale, Maria Woloshynowych, Martin Bland, Jeremy Miles, Ian Woods, Ann McEvoy, Donald Richardson, Glen Miller, Caroline Mosely, Dawn Taylor, Mary Nannary, and Sally Grabham. We are also grateful to clinical and administrative staff of the host hospital for their support.

On this paper there is acknowledgement of help from non-authors ...

Contributors: AB-AS designed and managed the project, wrote the research proposal, collected and analysed data, and wrote the final paper. TAS supervised the project; commented on the protocol, data collection, and analysis; was responsible for the quality control; and assisted on the paper. AC and AT piloted the instruments and process, assisted with stage two case note review, provided advice, and commented on the paper. Celia Grant, Eileen Richardson, William Gray, Yvonne Dobson, and Lorraine Wright screened the medical records and collected data in stage one and discussed the findings. AB-AS is the guarantor.

... as well as details about each author's contribution.

FIGURE 5.2   Another extract from a research paper from the *BMJ*; as well as details about each author's contribution, this time there is acknowledgement of help from non-authors.

surprisingly limited understanding and skill concerning the design and viability of a project. We found that there were times when we had to trust our own judgement (or should have done so) when it was out of keeping with the advice received from such seniors. The principle here is a simple one: avoid excessive reverence for senior researchers and accept nothing from them in an unquestioning way. Some enlightened senior researchers are fully aware of this risk, as the extract in Figure 5.3 shows.

> *It then dawned on me that experts like me commit two sins that retard the advance of science and harm the young. Firstly, adding our prestige to our opinions gives the latter far greater persuasive power than they deserve on scientific grounds alone. Whether through deference, fear, or respect, others tend not to challenge them, and progress towards the truth is impaired in the presence of an expert.*
>
> David Sackett, 2000

FIGURE 5.3   On avoiding too much reverence for senior researchers ...

Clinical collaborator

Unless you are already a senior clinician you will need a clinical ally for the project. This person is likely to be at a managerial level in the service and the sort of person who can allow use of health service facilities, sanction your use of time, and agree to the approach to patients or their records. He or she will probably be needed later when you apply formally for various kinds of permission to proceed (Chapter 16).

Most importantly, should you plan to carry out your field work in a clinical area where you are not already completely at home, this clinical collaborator (or a second one) will be your liaison with the service where you will collect your data. He or she might approach senior doctors or nurses, say, who will need to agree to have you around the Unit – or perhaps arrange for you to receive routine data from the records department.

Dinesh

We have already met Dinesh, an emergency department nurse. He is hoping to apply in due course for a health service research fellowship; if successful in the competition for such a secondment, he will be salaried at his current level for three or four years while he undertakes his project and completes a thesis for a PhD research degree. He needs to submit a proposed project and he has been working on a plan concerning an advocacy service for people who attend hospital because of self-harm. He has approached one of the academic psychiatrists, someone who carries out consultations in the emergency department, to ask whether she would supervise his application – and the project, if he is awarded the fellowship. The psychiatrist responded eagerly because these fellowships are seen in the academic community as prestigious; to be supervisor of someone holding such an award benefits the supervisor as well as the researcher.

She is already providing Dinesh with support and expertise but, although she is called regularly to the emergency department to provide senior psychiatric consultations, she isn't a member of the department's staff. Dinesh is going to need a senior person from the emergency department itself if he is to make much progress with his plan. The two of them arrange to meet with the clinical manager of the emergency department to discuss the evolving research idea and its needs. They find him very receptive and well aware that the service offered to people who attend after self-harm, especially after self-cutting, needs improvement. He will work to get acceptance from the clinical team for an advocacy service to function in the department. But first, he recognises that Dinesh will need to collect preliminary data about attendance patterns and numbers. He is going to arrange for Dinesh to gain access to the emergency department's computerised record system to collect these data, essential for the planning of the project.

Specialist assistance

All projects planned by new researchers will need the help of someone who has expertise in the science of research methods – research methodology. One or more persons on the team will need some expertise in epidemiology if you plan, for instance, a cohort analytic study or a case-control study. Alternatively, if the study is going to be based around interviews with patients who are to be invited to talk about their experience of receiving healthcare, someone must know about the design and conduct of qualitative research. Of course, in either case, this someone might be your supervisor, or it might be you – especially if you have had some research training and you can call on occasional advice from experts in these methods.

Statistical help is another common need, as is assistance from a librarian with expertise in systematic reviewing. Help from health economists, clinical trials units, and ethicists are more specialist requirements.

Dinesh and Anna

Dinesh, as his ideas for research develop into a definite project, is not looking as if he will need specialist help. His supervisor has considerable experience in basic clinical epidemiology and will be able to provide the advice required for the study design, data collection and analysis. For her project, however, Anna is going to need a supervisor who has specialist understanding of qualitative methods of research; either that or she and her supervisor will need additional help from such a person. She will need advice and practical help over a number of matters: whether to choose to undertake individual qualitative interviews or a group process (such as a focus group); how to go about taping and transcribing the interview or group interaction (getting the audio recording of the interview or focus group typed on to paper and a word-processed computer file – ready for analysis); and what method of qualitative questioning and analysis is best suited to the question and to the levels of skills and facilities available to her. She might be well advised to contact her nearest academic unit of primary care to see whether there is expertise available there along these lines. It might be that she will locate some useful supervision from someone who can help her through the design and planning of such practical steps as funding, permission, recording and transcribing, and so on. But she and the supervisor may need to approach another colleague who is a recognised qualitative expert – to establish the detailed design and to guide the analysis of the data.

Service users

It is becoming normal practice in health research for patients, clients, carers, and other representatives of the public who use the health service to be involved in research, not only as the subjects of study, as once was the case. Instead, researchers are realising that users of the service ought to take part in the setting up and the conduct of research – and influence the dissemination of the findings when they become available. Those who fund health research increasingly demand this process, and the research community is discovering how it adds value to all stages of the work of the researcher. This Patient and Public Involvement (PPI) might result in patients or service users advising on a research project, assisting in the project's design, maybe being employed as data-collecting researchers.

Service users contribute in four main ways to research. First, they may suggest improvements to the way that explanatory information and consent procedures are set out – checking their clarity and acceptability. Second, they may make useful suggestions concerning which outcomes and other measures might be important. Third, service users may propose alterations to design that take more account than you have of the expected experience of participants – perhaps there are going to be too many inconvenient appointments, or interviews will be too long, or too many blood samples are proposed. Fourth, in the timing of research participation, patient representatives can help point towards optimal times when interviews or other procedures might best be carried out when these occasions have to fit around treatments or hospital visits; for example, when would be the best time to interview parents of pre-term babies? Probably not when their baby is still in the hospital and the parents feel the need to be at the cot-side.

PPI representatives will frequently be members of funding committees (Chapter 15); they will expect research proposals to show suitable involvement of patients either as consultants or as collaborators. There are many sources of useful information about this increasingly important topic, see for example Figure 5.4.

INVOLVE: a health service-funded organisation (funded by the NIHR, the National Institute for Health Research) that promotes public involvement in NHS, public health and social care research.
www.invo.org.uk/

InvoNET: a network of people working to build evidence, knowledge and learning about public involvement in NHS, public health and social care research – part of the INVOLVE web site.
www.invo.org.uk/invoNET.asp

People in Research: a collaboration between INVOLVE and academic, charitable, commercial and government organisations.
http://www.peopleinresearch.org/

NHS Evidence – patient and public involvement: a specialist collection of NHS library materials about patients, users, carers, and the public in services – but includes links to information about research.
www.library.nhs.uk/PPI/

FIGURE 5.4   Some UK sources of information written for UK researchers – but with wider relevance, about public and patient involvement in research.

Anna

Anna has been giving thought to the process of patient and public involvement in her study. The practice already has a patient group – largely there to deal with matters related to the services provided. She reckons that she will be able to tap into existing eagerness among the actively involved patients in the group to help to shape her research idea. There is a maternity services arm to the practice's patient group, which may be the place to start discussions. She is thinking of contacting the person in her region who organises a support and pressure group for children believed to be damaged by vaccines. She will be discussing this possible step with senior colleagues in the practice as well as her research supervisor before going ahead; the sensitivities required for that contact will be greater than those associated with approaches towards parents in the practice.

You should now have assembled a team of helpers, each of them as eager as you to answer the proposed study question. Now you need to decide on the design of your study – the topic of the next chapter.

III

Get Set

6

Choosing the Best Study Design

Before going on in this chapter to tackle the choice of design, we have to make a declaration of our own interest in the matter of training. We three authors are heavily involved in introductory research training for healthcare professionals and research students. Some years back we decided that, in our experience of the health service and the medical school, there was far too little formal teaching about what is involved in a research project. We noticed that, in clinical practice, one would not set someone early in their career to undertake such procedures or treatments as minimally invasive surgery, cardiac catheterisation or dynamic psychotherapy – unless that person was first offered training, followed by supervision. But with research we found a different story: many newcomers to the task were expected to work out for themselves what to do, with little prior education about research. We also found that undergraduate programmes in medicine, nursing and the allied health professions, generally speaking, had offered little useful training in research skills.

For more than a decade we have therefore run a part-time postgraduate programme in health research that brings early-career health researchers together with other health professionals in our locality who are interested in undertaking research but have not yet started out. We find a steady stream of interest in attending and a keen appetite in the class for basic instruction in the relevant knowledge and skills. We cannot stress too forcefully our view: that you should try hard to find if there is such a programme available somewhere near you.

WHAT ARE THE RESEARCH DESIGN OPTIONS?

Quantitative methods

A new quantitative clinical research project is likely to be one of the following: a cross-sectional study (one- or two-group), a one-group longitudinal study, an ecological study, a case-control study, a cohort analytic study (retrospective or prospective), or a clinical trial (although a trial is unlikely to be suitable for an early-career researcher unless planned by an experienced trials researcher). It won't be at all easy to decide which design to choose unless you are reasonably familiar with these (and some other) options.

The study types set out above are pretty much the standard diet when it comes to the design components of quantitative health research. This present book is not the place to rehearse this material in detail; were we to do so we would need to keep it too short to do the topics justice. Instead, we will recommend here several best-selling books – all are good in their way, some longer and some shorter; all of them are ones that we like. Figure 6.1 is an illustrative example from our own book, *Understanding Clinical Papers* (Bowers *et al.*, 2006), in which there are three chapters about design of quantitative studies.

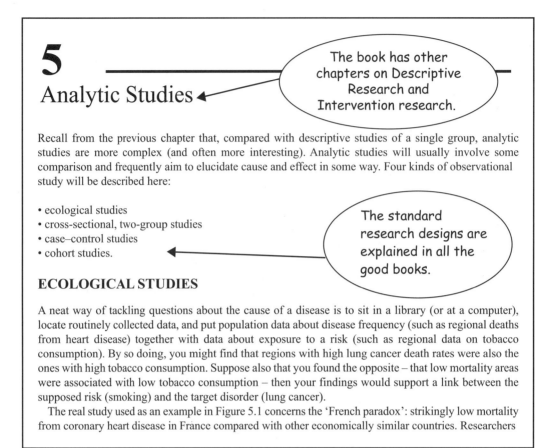

FIGURE 6.1 The architecture of research: a pointer towards three chapters about quantitative research design in our book *Understanding Clinical Papers* (Bowers, House and Owens, 2006).

We also recommend alternative books, all of which contain suitable accounts of the structure of quantitative clinical research. The chapters suggested here are the ones we think most relevant but there are many other useful chapters in these informative books: Bonita, Beaglehole and Kjellstrom, 2006, Chapter 3; Gordis (2008), Chapters 7–10; Hennekens and Buring (1987), Chapters 2, 5–8; Reigelman (2005), Section I: Chapters 2–12; Streiner and Norman (1998), Chapter 3.

In later chapters in this present book we present further material on sampling and analysis of quantitative studies.

QUALITATIVE METHODS

A qualitative project is likely to be undertaken by some form of non-participant observation, or through in-depth interviewing of individual people (most probably using some kind of purposive, quota or snowball sampling), or through the use of one or more focus groups. And for the gathering of the data and the plan for their analysis, the health researcher will probably be choosing between a grounded approach, a framework or thematic analysis, an interpretative phenomenological analysis, or some kind of content analysis.

As above, it will be necessary to know something of the design of qualitative research studies – as well as about sampling, collection and analysis – if a suitable design is to be set up in order to answer the research question. Once again, this book isn't the place for us to deal in detail with these techniques (although there is more later in the book on sampling and analysis). We recommend the following texts for an introduction. The chapters suggested here are the ones we think most relevant but there are many other useful chapters in these informative books: Pope and Mays (2006), Chapters 1–4; Ritchie and Lewis (2003), Chapters 3 and 4; Silverman (2005), Chapters 4, 8, 9.

DECIDING ON HOW THE QUESTION POINTS TOWARDS THE DESIGN

One of the main design decisions will be whether the question should be answered using qualitative or quantitative methods. Of course, a project might contain elements of both – a so-called mixed methods design – but it will be more straightforward here to consider the designs one at a time.

Suppose your research question concerned short stature in childhood and the potential for increasing adult height with the use of growth hormone. There are a number of questions about the amount of height gain that are likely to be tackled using quantitative methods. Whether growth hormone injections are effective in increasing growth velocity and final height in adulthood might be the target of clinical trials. Whether growth hormone has any adverse effects in the long term might be the target of cohort studies; growth hormone is such a rare form of prescribed medication that case-control studies are an unlikely choice of design. For the same reason, ecological designs are unlikely to be of great value. There is often a place for well-conducted cross-sectional quantitative designs. For example, determining the glucose tolerance among young people receiving growth hormone injections is likely to be a cross-sectional study; it may or may not be sensible to include a comparison group.

There is a parallel set of questions to be answered when qualitative rather than quantitative methods might be more useful. What does it feel like to hit early adulthood with short stature? What are the perceived effects on daily life? Is growth hormone injection delivered over many years an acceptable form of treatment? If there is early response and growth, promising much, but followed later by slowing (or even early cessation) of growth – how do people evaluate the benefits and downsides of the treatment programme? These questions could all be undertaken in a survey form – once or repeatedly – with quantitative analysis of the surveys. For example, the findings might be represented as proportions of people in various bands of expression of more or less satisfaction. There may well, however, be more of value to be gained from a qualitative rather than questionnaire approach: interviews with a relatively small number of patients, probing for their views on the target questions, going on with more participants until the same responses recur. These interviews might be undertaken individually or in groups. The methods described for eliciting the participants' responses vary greatly, as do the methods for analysing the material produced – which will usually be audio-recorded and transcribed on to paper word-for-word for the analysis stage.

Put another, simplistic, way – how much height gain can be achieved is a prime quantitative question, but the value of that gain, set against the drawbacks of the treatment, points towards a qualitative project.

Dinesh

You will recall that Dinesh was unhappy about the current care for people who have attended the emergency department because of an episode of self-harm, and he began to plan a research project to investigate the impact of a new advocacy service for these patients. He established through his search (Chapter 2) and his initial plan of action (Chapter 3) that he was thinking about some kind of before-and-after study: finding out about how advocacy might change someone's care – perhaps even in a clinical trial. His thoughts about measuring the effect of an advocacy service are about speed of repetition of self-harm and measures of mood before and after advocacy. It certainly seems that he is settling on a quantitative study design.

He has already seen (in Chapter 5) the need for epidemiological expertise but he has not yet finalised his decision about opting for cross-sectional, cohort or clinical trial design. It is time to make that choice. He has met with senior staff in the emergency department and with his own supervisor. They have discussed the design of the proposed study and they agreed that a clinical trial would be the definitive way of showing whether people who received an advocacy service repeated less often or not as soon, than those who received only the present form of care. They also agreed, with regret, that such a research study would be beyond their current resources. A clinical trial (a randomised controlled trial) would need many participants taking part in it in order to get a clear outcome, and Dinesh doesn't have time, money or experience for such an ambitious project.

If a clinical trial were to be planned – say for an application to a funding body – the researchers applying for a grant would need to make calculations about the numbers of participants needed. The researchers would need to specify the measures that they would use, and to predict confidently the numbers of patients who could be recruited from the emergency department. Dinesh and his senior colleagues decide that he should undertake a descriptive study aimed at gathering the data that would be needed *were* a clinical trial to be seriously proposed. He will collect data about the numbers and characteristics of patients attending the emergency department because of self-harm. He will follow them up through their medical records to establish the rate of repetition of self-harm – which may differ according to characteristics such as age or the method used in self-harm (poisoning or cutting, for example). He is also contemplating asking some of the patients who might be suited to entering a trial whether they would be willing to take part if, hypothetically, a trial of advocacy were to take place. He will also test out some measures of mood and of satisfaction with the care received.

Anna

Anna is plainly going down the qualitative research route. From the start of her deliberations about MMR injections she was intrigued by parents' apparent reluctance to bring their children for the vaccination. It seems likely that reluctance will be a complex matter, not readily measured by some scale nor explained by any numerical scoring. She has already settled, rather vaguely so far, on interviewing parents but she hasn't decided how this will be tackled: might she get a group of parents together, or would it work better were parents to be interviewed separately?

She has now established a link with her local academic unit of primary care and has been meeting with one of the staff there who has agreed to supervise. Anna and her supervisor have each found in their clinical practice that feelings run high, and they think that parents with opposing views might be challenging to handle in the group setting. Although it might be that well-run focus groups would be the most effective way to set about determining the factors that influence decisions about MMR vaccination, Anna is inexperienced in group work and her supervisor cannot spare the time to be there. Together they have decided that *individual face-to-face interviews* are likely to be more successful than a focus group.

Anna's next task, with her supervisor's help, will be to decide on which qualitative strategy her research will be based. She already knows from her clinical practice quite a lot about parents' feelings regarding MMR so she decides not to use a grounded theory approach. She considers interpretative phenomenological analysis (IPA) – which she and supervisor regard as potentially well suited to this question. Anna, however, has misgivings about her own psychological expertise and she thinks that IPA might prove demanding for someone with neither formal psychology training nor experience of the interpretations involved. She decides to opt for a semi-structured interview, with a pre-prepared topic guide (see Chapter 9), audio-taping each interview and transcribing the conversation. She plans to employ a thematic analysis searching the transcripts for the emerging themes that seem important when trying to describe the parents' decision-making about vaccination.

The next two chapters consider how researchers (including Dinesh and Anna) tackle the selection of study populations and study samples – in both quantitative and qualitative research.

7

Selecting Samples for Quantitative Research

In Chapter 6, you decided on the design of your study. You now need to start thinking about how you are going to get some subjects for your research. How you recruit your research subjects depends a lot on whether your research is going to be quantitative or qualitative (although the two methods can be used collaboratively, and often are). In this chapter we will look at the quantitative research case, but regardless of your approach there are several issues which you need to consider.

WHICH SUBJECTS? – THE SAMPLE

- Who or what will be your research subjects? Will they be people – for example, patients, or individuals drawn from the general population? Or things – for instance, swabs, slides, tissue samples, wound dressings, and so on?
- How many subjects will you need, that is, what size of sample?
- How will you select your subjects?
- Who will you want to include in your sample, and who will you need to exclude?
- Finally, whatever you discover about your particular sample, will you want to be able to generalise your findings to a wider population?

As for the last question, you are almost certain to want to generalise your results if your research is to be quantitative, but not necessarily if qualitative. In this chapter we are going to deal with the quantitative case (except for the sample size question which we will examine in Chapter 10), and in the next chapter the qualitative case.

THE STUDY AND TARGET POPULATIONS

In statistics we think of a population as any complete *set* of items or individuals. You, the researcher, define the population you want to study. For example, if you are based in a Glasgow hospital and want to investigate the risk factors for low birthweight babies, you might define your population as every low-birthweight baby born in Glasgow, or in Scotland. Or more ambitiously, in the UK.

We call such a population a *target* population. As you can imagine, identifying and listing every member of any target population is usually impossible. For this reason we usually have to lower our sights a little and work instead with what is known as the *study* population. The study population is a more accessible

Getting Started in Health Research, First Edition. David Bowers, Allan House and David Owens.
© 2011 David Bowers, Allan House and David Owens. Published 2011 by Blackwell Publishing Ltd.

subset of the target population. You will select the group of subjects you will actually work with (the sample) from the study population. There are two important questions:

- First, how representative of the study population is the sample?
- And second, how representative of the target population is the study population?

The meaning of your research findings in the wider arena will depend on the degree of this representativeness. As we noted above, the ability to generalise is usually less important for the qualitative researcher, but nonetheless needs to be borne in mind.

GETTING YOUR SAMPLE SUBJECTS WHEN YOUR RESEARCH IS QUANTITATIVE

Now is a good time to write down the answers to these two questions:

- What exactly is your target population?
- What study population is available to you?

Make sure that your descriptions are as detailed as possible, with a note of all the characteristics of the subjects you wish to study in your research. After you have read the discussion which follows you will need to decide which method of collecting your own sample is both appropriate and feasible.

PROBABILITY SAMPLING

The most representative sample is the random sample, also known as a probability sample, in which your subjects are selected at random from the population. The main types of probability sampling methods are outlined below. You should read through this now, but bear in mind that this is not a statistics textbook. Before you embark on any research project, you should expect to have to do a lot of preliminary reading, and this will include material on sampling and other statistical procedure. If, as will usually be the case, you are not able to take a random sample, a reasonable compromise is often consecutive or contact sampling (we describe this shortly).

- *Simple random sampling*. To take a simple random sample, every member of the population is identified and listed (this list is called a sample frame), and from this list a sample of the required size is selected using, for example, a table of random numbers, or a computer programme that generates random numbers.
- *Systematic random sampling*. Subjects are chosen at regular intervals from the sampling frame, until the desired sample size is achieved. For example, if you want a sample of 100 from a population of 1500, then you select every 15th (1500/100) subject, until you get 100. The first one to be selected is determined by selecting a number from 1 to 15 randomly.
- *Stratified random sampling*. If you want to ensure that some smaller sections of your population are not missed out of your sample, for example a minority ethnic group, then you can divide the sample frame into strata, based on ethnicity, and sample randomly from each of these strata, in proportion to the share of each ethnic group in the population as a whole.
- *Cluster sampling*. Suppose you were investigating some aspect of the treatment of diabetic patients in England. Your target population is all diabetic patients in England (the patients would be your study

units). Realistically, it would be impossible to construct a sampling frame for this large population, however you can proceed as follows:

(a) Define diabetic *clinics* as your study units – in each of which there will be a '*cluster*' of patients.

(b) List all of these clusters in your region – let's say there are 25 (this is your study population).

(c) You can then take a random sample of say five clinics from this list (maybe systematically), and select all eligible patients in these five clinics. This then is your sample.

• *Multistage cluster sampling.* Cluster sampling but with more than one stage.

The big advantage of cluster sampling is that we don't need a complete sample for the individual study units – which as we have mentioned already is usually impossible.

For an illustration of cluster sampling see Figure 7.1. This is from a study of the quality of life of Swedish children with asthma.

CHILDREN
Asthma – quality of life for Swedish children

Ingela Rydström, Ann-Charlotte Dalheim-Englund, Birgit Holritz-Rasmussen, Christian Möller and Per-Olof Sandman

---

The basis for this prospective cross-sectional survey was all hospitals in Sweden with a specialist clinic (n = 67) where children with asthma are treated. Of these, 15 clinics (based on a power analysis) were randomly selected and invited to participate in the study. The allergy nurse at each of the selected clinics consecutively contacted 20 children with asthma and their parents, who visited the clinic for an asthma-related check up and asked them to complete a questionnaire (PAQLQ) about their experiences of QoL.

There are 67 hospitals in Sweden with specialist asthma clinics. These clinics formed the 67 clusters...

... from which 15 clinics were randomly selected ......

... and from each of these 20 children were consecutively contacted, to give 300 study units (300 children).

FIGURE 7.1 An example of cluster sampling from a quality of life study for children with asthma.

As you can see, the original study unit is the asthma clinic. Each of the 67 asthma clinics is a *cluster* of children with asthma, so there are 67 clusters. 15 of these clusters are randomly selected,[1] and 20 children consecutively selected from each of these clusters. These 300 children now become the study units.

If your sample will be made up not of people but items (plasma samples, biopsy tissue, etc.), then random sampling may well be possible, because it will often be easier to construct a sample frame with such populations.

---

[1] The decision to select 15 clinics is based on the sample size required to meet the power calculation. We discuss the sample size issue in Chapter 10.

NON-PROBABILISTIC SAMPLING

In theory, probabilistic sampling methods of the types described above are to be preferred. However, in practice less rigorous, *non*-probabilistic methods often have to be employed in clinical research. One of the most common is consecutive sampling, which we discuss now.

CONSECUTIVE SAMPLING

In this approach the sample subjects may be selected from individuals who have some contact with your department or clinic, for example your last (or next) 100 consecutive patients, or all of the patients you saw last year. Such samples clearly do not need a sampling frame. The samples recruited this way can, with care, be reasonably representative. To illustrate this idea, Figure 7.2 is an extract from a study into the use of azithromycin for acute bronchitis. As you can see, the subjects were selected on the basis of clinical contact.

Azithromycin for acute bronchitis: a randomised, double-blind, controlled trial

Arthur T Evans, Shahid Husain, Lakshmi Durairaj, Laura S Sadowski, Marjorie Charles-Damte, Yue Wang

---

Methods
Participants
After approval of the study protocol by the institutional review board, we recruited adult patients without chronic lung disease who presented with cough of 2–14 days duration and were diagnosed with acute bronchitis by attending physicians in the adult ambulatory screening clinic of Cook County Hospital, during weekdays from December 1999 until March 2000.

FIGURE 7.2   An example of consecutive sampling in a study of azithromycin for acute bronchitis. In all 220 subjects were recruited.

In contact sampling we could also include samples where the subjects are drawn from a clinical *registry* or *database*, established from previous clinical contacts. In some cases these may provide a decent sampling frame. Figure 7.3 is an example where researchers in a case-control study of semen quality in survivors of childhood cancer used a clinical database. This database will clearly *not* contain information on *all* childhood survivors of cancer in Edinburgh or in Scotland, but may be reasonably representative of this population.

CONVENIENCE SAMPLING

In addition to consecutive sampling, researchers will sometimes use a sample which is convenient for them. Such as a group of students, or some of their colleagues, or one day's worth of clinic patients. They know that these samples are unlikely to be representative of any population they may have in mind, but may be useful for road-testing an idea, or a questionnaire, or helpful in a pilot study.

Semen quality and spermatozoal DNA integrity in survivors of childhood cancer: a case-control study

Angela B Thomson, Alastair J Campbell, D Stewart Irvine, Richard A Anderson, Christopher JH Kelnar, Dr W Hamish B Wallace

Patients

We searched the oncology database at the Royal Hospital for Sick Children, Edinburgh, for all male survivors of childhood cancer aged older than 16 years, and identified 51 individuals between December 1999 and June 2001.

Figure 7.3   An example of the use of a database from a case-control study into semen quality in survivors of childhood cancer.

Finally, note that research studies that reach out to the population are often referred to as population-based studies. Population-based studies may also recruit individuals by means of posters and leaflets placed in health centres or circulated to healthcare workers, or through media publicity campaigns (local newspapers and radio stations), or through random telephone dialling, and so on.

Dinesh

Having given some thought to the issues raised above, Dinesh refines his questions about the people he wants to study (Figure 7.4).

SELECTING CONTROLS FOR A CASE-CONTROL STUDY

If you have chosen to do a case-control study then you will also need to decide where and how you are going to recruit your control subjects. Controls can be matched or unmatched, but either way, the general idea is that the controls should be selected from the same population as your cases, so that any differences between the two groups is likely to be related to the fact that one group (cases) has the condition that you are interested in while the other (the controls) doesn't. The challenge is that, despite your best efforts, your controls may differ in important ways from the cases, and this may well lead you to draw misleading conclusions from your study.

One way round this problem is to match for some obvious factors, such as age and sex. As an example, the controls in a study of the semen quality of childhood cancer survivors were matched only for age (they are of course necessarily all male) – see Figure 7.5.

A word of caution – be careful not to overmatch. For example, suppose you were planning a case-control study of the possibility of a relationship between obesity and breathlessness. If you matched for smoking status, as well as age and sex, how could your study show that it might be smoking which is the risk factor for breathlessness and not obesity? For this reason you should be cautious about matching on anything other than age and sex.

So, if you have chosen a case-control design, you need to decide on unmatched or matched controls – if the latter, what factors you intend to match on. You need to write this down as well as how you propose to recruit the controls. Note that getting suitable controls can often be difficult.

DINESH'S LIST OF QUESTIONS AND HIS THOUGHTS ON EACH

What's my target population?

I don't have any reason to suspect that the characteristics of self-harm patients will differ in different regions of the UK. So I'm going to make it all patients attending EDs in the UK after an episode of self-harm. Then I can generalise more widely.

What about my study population?

I've already decided to select subjects from my own ED, being the only one in the city (see Chapter 3), and it'll be a lot easier than selecting from EDs in other cities also. And anyway I don't think there is any substantial difference in the make-up of the patients at other EDs in the region.

How will I get my sample from my study population?

I'm going to use clinical records to measure stuff like throughput of patients, proportion re-attending within 6 months, drop-out rates, and so on. But for the other stuff (proportion consenting to an advocate, satisfaction, mood, access to patients, staff co-operation issues, etc.) I'm going to do a small prospective study, and need to think about how to select a sample.

Comparison group?

I'm doing a comprehensive prospective design so no comparison group.

My inclusion and exclusion criteria.

Inclusion: All adult pts presenting to my ED with self-harm. Exclusion: those who cannot consent..

Which variables do I want to measure?

Age, gender, type of s-h, history of s-h, mood, satisfaction (I want to pilot both a mood and a satisfaction scale).

FIGURE 7.4   Dinesh refines his questions about the people he wants to study.

Semen quality and spermatozoal DNA integrity in survivors of childhood cancer: a case-control study

Angela B Thomson, Alastair J Campbell, D Stewart Irvine, Richard A Anderson, Christopher JH Kelnar, Dr W Hamish B Wallace

For each study participant, we recruited two aged-matched controls (n = 66). The volunteers were recruited by advertisement in local media and through hospital outpatient clinics, and were selected on the basis of the absence of any clinical evidence, on history or physical examination, of reproductive health problems.

FIGURE 7.5   The selection of controls in a case-control study of semen quality in survivors of childhood cancer.

INCLUSION AND EXCLUSION CRITERIA

Before we leave sampling for quantitative research, you need to think about which subjects you want to include in your sample, and which, perhaps more particularly, to exclude. Here are two things for you to do:

- Write down a set of criteria defining precisely which subjects you want to include in your sample. These criteria will be dictated by your research objectives and the exact characteristics of the population you want to study (as well as by ethical considerations – more on the latter in Chapter 16).
- Write down a set of criteria which define the subjects you will need to exclude. For instance, patients with complications, or who are currently taking a drug, or who have another concurrent condition, or are pregnant, and so on. The detailed definition of your population you wrote earlier will help here.

As an example, Figure 7.6 is an extract from a study of methotrexate in rheumatoid arthritis, illustrating the inclusion and exclusion criteria used by the researchers.

HAVING GOT YOUR STUDY PARTICIPANTS HOW ARE YOU GOING TO GET THE DATA FROM THEM?

In quantitative research you will usually get your data for a number of variables:

- By measuring something. For example, diastolic blood pressure, or survival time.
- By counting something. For example, the number of pressure sores, or angina attacks, or abnormal cells.
- From the completion of a questionnaire or the use of a measuring scale. For example, a patient satisfaction questionnaire, or the Edinburgh Post-Natal Depression Scale.
- Observing something. For example, skin pallor, or stool quality.

As an example, in the study on methotrexate for rheumatoid arthritis referred to above, the researchers obtained data on 16 variables for 1240 subjects, both clinical and demographic (see Figure 7.7). In addition, patients were asked to respond to questions from an acute bronchitis 'Health-Related Quality of Life' questionnaire.

Methotrexate and mortality in patients with rheumatoid arthritis: a prospective study

Hyon K Choi, Miguel A Hernán, John D Seeger, James M Robins, Frederick Wolfe

Participants

We *included* in our analysis individuals who were older than 18 years and who attended the Wichita Arthritis Center at least twice between Jan 1, 1981 (when weekly low-dose methotrexate therapy and health assessment questionnaire score became available) and Dec 31, 1999; had rheumatoid arthritis fulfilling the 1958–87 American College of Rheumatology criteria for rheumatoid arthritis; and had not received methotrexate before their first visit to the center.

As in randomized trials assessing methotrexate, we *excluded* patients (irrespective of methotrexate exposure status) with any of the following contraindications for methotrexate use: pregnancy, expectation of pregnancy, heavy alcohol use, recent malignant disease, renal insufficiency, chronic liver disease, leukopenia, thrombocytopenia, and known non-compliance.

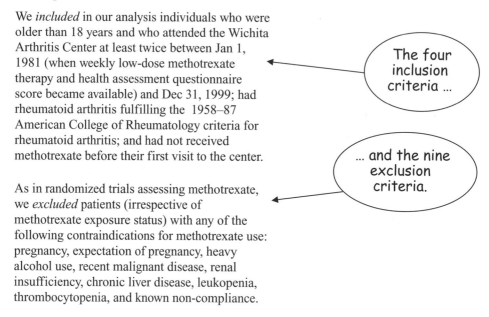

The four inclusion criteria …

… and the nine exclusion criteria.

FIGURE 7.6   Inclusion and exclusion criteria in a study of methotrexate and mortality in patients with rheumatoid arthritis (our italics).

Methotrexate and mortality in patients with rheumatoid arthritis: a prospective study

Hyon K Choi, Miguel A Hernán, John D Seeger, James M Robins, Frederick Wolfe

Methods

Study data

Since 1974, we have enrolled more than 2000 consecutive individuals with rheumatoid arthritis seen at the Wichita Arthritis Center, an outpatient rheumatology facility. We entered details of participants into a computerized database at the time of their first clinic visit, and obtained and added demographic (education level, smoking history, total income, and marital status), clinical (tender joint count, grip strength, morning stiffness, health assessment questionnaire disability index score, arthritis impact measurement scales, including depression scales, visual analogue scale for pain, visual analogue scale for patients' global assessment of disease status, and body mass index), laboratory (erythrocyte sedimentation rate, white blood cell counts, and concentrations of haemoglobin and rheumatoid factor), medication use, and self-reported data at each follow-up visit.

FIGURE 7.7   List of variables both clinical and demographic for which data was collected from 1240 subjects in a study of methotrexate and mortality in patients with rheumatoid arthritis.

Dinesh

Dinesh spends some time considering the best way for him to select a sample of the participants he will need for his research. The alternatives and his thoughts on these are shown in Figure 7.8.

- Consecutive sampling —— *Promising – I understand this and it should be fairly straightforward*

- Convenience sampling —— *People might avoid 'tricky' customers*

- Quota sampling

- Systematic sampling —— *My Thursday off? But benefits day?*

- Simple randomised sampling —— *How could I arrange that?*

- Stratified random sampling

- Multi-stage sampling

FIGURE 7.8   Dinesh considers different approaches to choosing his sample.

We will have a lot more to say on preparing to collect and measure data in Chapter 9, on recruiting participants in Chapter 17, and on the actual collection and recording of data in Chapter 18.

8

Selecting Samples for Qualitative Research

GETTING YOUR SAMPLE PARTICIPANTS – THE QUALITATIVE RESEARCH CASE

If you are a qualitative researcher you will often be less interested in recruiting a large representative (and thus generalisable) sample, and more interested in the selection of a possibly limited number of *information-rich* participants. These may have the potential to contribute the most to an understanding of how particular variables manifest themselves in certain groups of participants. Such participants, though, may not be typical of the wider population which is not as important if generalisability is not a priority. Note that these approaches are non-probabilistic (i.e. they are not based on random sampling procedures).

We can divide non-probability sampling methods into two broad types: convenient, or purposive. Most qualitative sampling methods are purposive in nature because we usually approach the sampling problem with a specific plan or purpose in mind. We have summarised the most common methods below, but you will need to do plenty of reading yourself (see, for example, Ritchie and Lewis, *Qualitative Research Practice*) and consult your mentor or supervisor, after which you will have to decide which method you think is appropriate in your case.

CONVENIENCE SAMPLES

Convenience samples (also known as availability, or haphazard samples) are samples that are selected because they are easily accessible by the researcher – there is no sampling strategy as such. For example, subjects may be members of your team, or a small group of willing patients, or volunteer first-year students, and so on. Their big advantage is that they are easy to recruit, but they are hardly likely to be representative of any particular population nor have the characteristics in which you are interested.

PURPOSIVE SAMPLING

There are a number of sampling methods that can be classified as purposive, but their common feature is that the researcher deliberately or purposely chooses subjects to represent types of individuals according to certain key criteria. These criteria will be based on a number of factors. For example, the main aims of the study, any hypotheses that the investigators want to explore, what might already be known about the research topic, or what might not be known. Here are a few examples to illustrate this idea.

Getting Started in Health Research, First Edition. David Bowers, Allan House and David Owens.
© 2011 David Bowers, Allan House and David Owens. Published 2011 by Blackwell Publishing Ltd.

Extreme case sampling

This method focuses on subjects who are unusual or special in some way. For example, patients who recover uncharacteristically quickly from some trauma, or some clinical intervention (or conversely those who recover very slowly). Or patients who are extremely poor at taking medication consistently. Or patients who experience an extreme reaction to a commonly used therapeutic procedure. Or patients who always have an extremely aggressive attitude towards clinical staff. Or patients who have extremely strong emotional reactions to some stimulus or experience. And so on.

Intense case sampling

Similar to extreme case sampling but not quite as extreme. The sample subjects manifest the phenomenon in question *intensely*, but not so extremely. They are still information-rich.

Maximum variation (or heterogeneous) sampling (also known as *sampling for diversity*)

A maximum variation sample will consist of subjects chosen with the purpose of ensuring that they collectively represent as wide a range as possible of variation in the factors considered relevant to the object of the study. For example, the treatment of epilepsy may be hindered by the stigma experienced by those with the illness. In order to obtain insight in how this phenomenon manifests itself in different ethnic cultures (say white versus Asian); or between males and females; or in rural versus urban areas; or in well-to-do and in economically deprived patients; or in those well-educated and those ill-educated, a researcher must ensure that all of these groups are included in the sample.

Homogeneous sampling

Selects a small sample having similar characteristics in order to describe some particular subgroup in depth. For example, the attitudes to their prospective newborns of husbands of women having IVF, or the health needs of immigrant agricultural workers.

Typical case sampling

Subjects are selected who are typical of the group of interest. For example, the health problems of the 'typical' young offender, or the mental health issues around the typical socially isolated female living in a particular ethnic community.

Critical case sampling

Looks for critical cases that can 'make the difference' dramatically. For example, you might have developed a new approach to encourage the use of contraceptives among men in rural communities in a developing country. You select a sample of men who are largely poor and illiterate, as 'test cases'. If this group is able to adopt the method successfully, then this provides some indication that it might be successful among the wider rural male population.

Snowball (or chain) sampling

Snowball sampling is especially useful when you are trying to reach populations that are inaccessible or hard to find. For example, suppose you want to investigate some aspect of the well-being of homeless intravenous drug users. If you could find one such person, you could ask him or her if they could tell you where you could find another such user. This next person might then be able to point you towards another user, and so on, and so on.

AN EXAMPLE OF MAXIMUM VARIATION SAMPLING (OR SAMPLING FOR DIVERSITY)

Researchers wanted to discover the views of patients about their discharge from outpatients clinics, whether these perceptions changed over time, and whether the discharge process could be improved for the patient. They described their method as shown in Figure 8.1.

Patients' views on their discharge from follow-up in outpatient clinics: qualitative study

Yvonne Burkey, Mary Black, Hugh Reeve

Methods

We identified 159 patients who had been followed up for some time (three or more attendances) at five general medical outpatient clinics, and had been discharged. We selected 52 of these patients to cover a range of experiences related to discharge -- men and women of different ages, attending a variety of clinics for different conditions. Patients who had been discharged by doctors of various grades were selected so that we could determine whether they considered that more senior doctors handled the discharge process better.

> 52 patients were selected from the original 159 so that they represented a wide variety of discharge experiences – both men and women, of differing ages, attending a variety of clinics, and so on.

Forty-three consenting patients were subsequently interviewed in their own homes within two weeks of discharge … One of us interviewed 15 patients in depth, using a topic guide to focus the discussion. Analysis of early transcripts showed that we had identified the range of themes and issues; we then developed a more structured schedule for the remaining 28 first interviews. These were undertaken by a trained qualitative interviewer.

Three months later, second interviews were conducted with 37 of the 45 patients (two had died and six withdrew). These interviews aimed to explore whether the patients' feelings about discharge had changed and to elicit their views on the care provided by their GP. All second interviews were semi-structured. They covered specific issues which had arisen for individual patients at the first interview and areas relevant to all patients.

All interviews were tape-recorded and were transcribed fully for analysis. Data from all the interviews were analysed qualitatively by reading and re-reading interview transcripts and schedules. This process enabled us to identify issues and themes.

FIGURE 8.1   A description of a maximum variation study.

THEORETICAL SAMPLING

This is a form of purposive sampling in which the researchers collect data which they feel might contribute to the development of a particular theory. The process is generally iterative in that the researchers analyse the data collected and then, in the light of their findings, collect a further sample to refine and develop the theory. This process continues until no new analytic insights are revealed. The selection criteria are founded on theoretical relevance and the theoretical purpose of the study.

HAVING GOT YOUR SAMPLE HOW ARE YOU GOING TO GET THE DATA FROM IT?

Whereas quantitative researchers will usually collect data by measuring (or counting), and they may also use closed-question questionnaires, qualitative researchers tend to rely less on measurement and more on:

- In-depth, open-ended individual face-to-face interviews. Data from these interviews may consist of direct quotations from people about their experiences, opinions and beliefs, feelings, ideas, knowledge, and so on.
- Focus groups. Similar to above but group responses. Data may be *summaries* of beliefs, attitudes, etc. as expressed by the group.
- Direct observation. This can provide detailed descriptions of people's behaviours, actions and interactions, etc. May be either individual or group.
- Written documents. For example, open-ended written items on questionnaires, diaries, correspondence, official reports, other written accounts, and so on.

To repeat, we will have a lot more to say on preparing to collect and measure data in Chapter 9, on recruiting participants in Chapter 17, and on the actual collection and recording of data in Chapter 18. In Chapter 22 we will discuss ways in which you can analyse and make sense of your results.

Anna

Anna is moving towards thinking that individual face-to-face interviews will be the way to go (see next chapter) but in any case now needs to decide which of the above sampling methods will be the most appropriate. Her thinking is shown in Figure 8.2.

So Anna decides to contact all those mothers on the practice list who have children under 12 months, either collaring them when they come to the surgery for any reason, or if they don't visit within a three-month period, by telephoning them. She hopes to be able to recruit enough mothers this way. She thinks, "when I've got my sample I will divide it into three groups: MMR mothers; single-jab mothers; no-jab mothers. This will ensure that I get adequate coverage of all three of these important jab categories."

Having decided on a method of selecting the participants for your research project, you want now to think about what information you will need to collect from them. We will deal with this question in the following chapter.

Convenience sampling?

This would mean taking as a sample only those mums who visit the surgery for any reason at all. But this won't do because I'm not going to get to see mums who don't come, which will include some of those who are MMR-reluctant. Looks like a purposive sample then.

Extreme-case or intense-case sampling?

This won't work because I can't identify those mums who have 'extreme' views on MMR until I've interviewed them! Vicious circle.

A maximum-variation sample?

I think this is the one I want. I'm anxious to include all the mums on my list, regardless of age, education, number of kids, previous MMR history, ethnicity, and so on. So I want as diverse a sample as poss. And this rules out homogeneous, typical case, and critical case samples, so I can forget about these.

FIGURE 8.2   Anna's thinking on possible sampling methods.

Wait for It

9

Deciding What Information to Collect

WHAT DO WE NEED TO KNOW?

Having decided who will be the participants in your research, the next question is – what information do you want to collect about or from them?

There are different reasons to collect information, and different ways of collecting it, and you will need to decide the details depending on your question and study design. However, a common starting place that is appropriate to most types of research is to record information that allows you to describe your sample.

The characteristics that define populations are often called *demographics* or *demographic data*, and the same term is conventionally used for characteristics that describe samples. Typical examples include age, sex, ethnicity and socio-economic status. Which other characteristics you record will depend on your study; the purpose of demographics is to allow your reader to interpret your findings knowing about the sample you studied. Thus you might record educational history, family structure, smoking or alcohol consumption. In clinical studies, researchers often record details of participants' health state – any disease they have, its stage severity and treatment. These are sometimes called *case-mix measures* for obvious reasons.

There are some differences in the approach to information-recording in quantitative compared to qualitative research. We will deal with each in turn.

RECORDING INFORMATION IN QUALITATIVE RESEARCH

The range of what is recorded in qualitative research is broad. Figure 9.1 illustrates some examples of what might be the focus of information collection in qualitative research.

- beliefs
- attitudes or opinions
- accounts of personal experiences
- personal explanations for or understandings of something
- interactions with somebody else; social behaviour
- non-verbal communications

FIGURE 9.1 Some examples of what might be the focus of information collection in qualitative research.

Getting Started in Health Research, First Edition. David Bowers, Allan House and David Owens.
© 2011 David Bowers, Allan House and David Owens. Published 2011 by Blackwell Publishing Ltd.

Anna

As Anna thinks about this, she realises that many of the items on this list may be relevant – beliefs about MMR and its risks and benefits; opinions about which of those risks or benefits matter most; personal experiences upon which those beliefs or opinions might be based and so on. She is also aware that in her GP work she can spot other clues about how people will respond to prompts to vaccinate their children – for example, their reliability in keeping appointments, the way they talk to receptionists, and the way they behave with their children during consultations. She has to choose which of all these possibilities to concentrate on, and because this is her first research project she opts for something simple. She will try and identify mothers' beliefs and opinions about MMR, and any personal experiences that have formed those ideas.

Next, Anna needs to decide how to collect the relevant information. She has a look in an introductory textbook and discovers there are several ways to go about this – shown in Figure 9.2.

The List	Anna's thoughts
Send a questionnaire	Lots of people won't respond. Anyway, not sure how to design it.
Make observations about responses during consultations	Too complicated for my first project.
Ask mums to write down their thoughts	Likely low response. Will miss those with literacy problems.
Hold a focus group	Don't know how to run one! Will mums speak freely in front of others?
Interview mothers face to face	This is most like what I do every day anyway. Plays to my strengths.

FIGURE 9.2   Anna's list of possible approaches to information-gathering and her thoughts about each.

In the end Anna thinks that the most successful approach will be to do face-to-face interviews with the mothers (parents), to explore with them the reasons why they made the decision that they did. (This is the same approach she considered a possibility in her initial plan of action – see Chapter 3.)

Anna wants to conduct a non-threatening fairly open interview in which she explores parents' thinking. She has done some reading and knows that she still has to standardise the interview so that all participants discuss all the areas in which she is interested. Rather than a list of fixed questions she needs a *topic guide*. From her thinking about her question (see Chapter 2) she decides she will make a provisional list of topics she will need to cover in at least the areas shown in Figure 9.3.

So, Anna's conclusion is that she will conduct individual face-to-face interviews with her mothers, using a pre-prepared topic guide to explore their beliefs and opinions about MMR and the personal experiences that have influenced those ideas.

Now that Anna has decided the type of data she wants to collect, she will need to decide the exact method she will use to capture those data. For most types of data – even in qualitative research – there is more than one way

- First some questions about the family
    - Mother and partner
    - Children and their ages
    - All children current partner's?
    - How does childcare work?
    - Who tends to make childcare decisions?

- The history of immunisation in the family
    - Previous children – all treated the same?
    - Youngest child - same as others or different?
        - if different why?
    - Any children had infectious diseases?
        - if so, immunised or not?

- Information and opinions about MMR
    - Sources of information (family, friends, professionals)
    - Which source most valued

- Possible outcomes mum associates with immunisations
    - MMR and others
    - Good and bad outcomes
    - Reasons for expectations
    - Family experience, magazine articles, etc.

FIGURE 9.3   Anna's provisional topic guide.

to do this. For example:

Observations – notes taken by observer or interviewer
Interview notes – written comments made at the time or later
Audio or video recording – usually transcribed later.

Anna decides that although she usually just makes her own notes when interviewing patients, she may miss important pieces of information if she does that. She will also not be able to get help from a collaborator in exploring the women's answers. So she decides to audiotape the interviews and arrange to have them transcribed, so that she can re-read for new ideas and also share with collaborators if possible.

RECORDING INFORMATION IN QUANTITATIVE RESEARCH

The main challenge in quantitative research is to collect information in a measurable form, and to use a measure that is accurate. (For further discussion of the characteristics of measures, you might like to consult our companion text, *Understanding Clinical Papers* (Bowers *et al.*, 2006).) Let's use as an example what Dinesh decides to do about measuring *mood* in his research.

Dinesh

Dinesh writes down a list of characteristics of a desirable measure (see Figure 9.4).

Dinesh's list	Dinesh's notes
Is the content what I'm interested in?	I need to check combined depression <u>and</u> anxiety measures
Are the specific questions <u>good</u> <u>at</u> picking up the content I want?	Is this what people mean by <u>validity</u>?
Is the measure reliable – will it get the same result every time I use it?	I know this one – it's repeatability or <u>reliability</u>
Is the measure going to pick up changes over time, between groups?	Check <u>sensitivity to change</u>
It's got to be acceptable	Quick and easy to use, understandable, readily available, usable by a wide range of people

FIGURE 9.4   Dinesh's notes about choice of measure.

With this checklist, Dinesh can go away and check what's available off the shelf. He consults textbooks (including some recommended by a psychiatric colleague), asks a librarian to help him search for widely used measures, and looks to see what's been used in other studies. His line of thinking (correctly) is that it's far better to use an existing measure than to make one up of his own – its characteristics are likely to have been properly established, its usefulness and drawbacks will be clear, and it will allow him to compare his findings directly with those of other people. The particular measure he chooses will depend upon the trade-offs between these various characteristics – for example, a very short measure (i.e. a measure with only a small number of questions) may be simple and quick but not cover all the content he wants.

One other consideration in choice of measures may be cost – some standardised measures are copyrighted by commercial publishing companies whilst others are in the public domain. Dinesh's list of measures now looks as shown in Figure 9.5.

When Dinesh thinks about the methods he might use to capture these data he comes up with three methods:

- Emergency department computer system – attendances
  - methods of self-harm
- Patient records – clinical assessment
- Patient-completed questionnaires – mood (PHQ9)
  - satisfaction.

SETTING	City population Annual attendances (all) Annual attendances (self-harm)
SAMPLE	Number Age (mean, range) Methods used (adopt standard system used by other researchers)
ASSESSMENT	List routinely collected clinical data (Emergency Dept proforma)
INTERVENTION	Narrative account of the work done by peer mentors (including training and supervision)
OUTCOMES	- Time to re-presentation - Reason for re-presentation (adopt standard categories used by other researchers) - Questionnaire for mood (PHQ9) - Satisfaction with service (still need to find good measure)

FIGURE 9.5   Dinesh's provisional list of measures.

By now you should have a clear idea of the research design you will use, the sample you will study, what data you will collect and how. The next thing that you might want to do is think about how to organise and analyse your data once you have collected them. But before we get to that topic we need to think about two further aspects of design – one of which only applies to quantitative research (planning to tackle confounders), and the other of which applies to all research (deciding on sample size). We will deal with these issues in the next two chapters.

10

Tackling Confounders

INTRODUCTION

In Chapter 9 you listed the variables that you want to study. In this chapter we want to discuss the concept of *confounding* – a problem which often arises when the possible relationships between a number of variables are being studied. Confounding is only really a problem if your research is *quantitative.*

To illustrate, supposing a research team were investigating the potential benefits of hormone replacement therapy (HRT): imagine that they observe, in a cohort analytic study, that women who were taking HRT developed fewer heart attacks than did women of the same age who had not been taking HRT. Suppose also that those women in the study who were prescribed HRT were financially better off, smoked less, exercised more, and ate a diet with more fruit and vegetables and less fat. It is immediately clear that, although the observation that the women who took HRT had less heart disease was true, the explanation might be due to these other influences rather than any protection from the HRT. These other influences are the *confounding variables* or *confounders.*

In this chapter, we are going to look at:

- What confounding is
- Some ways in which it can be dealt with.

This chapter is going to be rather more technical than most others in the book so far, because getting a grasp of confounding is so important at the design stage of quantitative research. We provide an introduction to the problem and suggest a few ways of dealing with it. We will return to the subject in Chapter 21, where we will discuss further procedures for dealing with confounding.

CONFOUNDING – WHAT IS IT?

Suppose you notice that people's hair colour seems to be associated with frequency of heart attacks. In particular, the more grey hair people have, the greater the frequency of heart attacks. If you were naive you might conclude that having grey hair is a cause of heart attacks. Of course this is nonsense. The true relationship is between *age* and heart attacks – it is being older that is the relevant factor here, not hair colour.

Looking at the proposition concerning grey hair and heart disease in more detail, suppose that you carried out a cohort study in which you followed up people with clearly grey hair and determined how many (what proportion) of them had a heart attack over the next five years; you do the same with a

Getting Started in Health Research, First Edition. David Bowers, Allan House and David Owens.
© 2011 David Bowers, Allan House and David Owens. Published 2011 by Blackwell Publishing Ltd.

comparison group who have little or no grey hair at the start of the study. You find that incidence of heart attack is much greater among the grey-hair group. At first sight 'exposure' to the risk factor of having grey hair appears to be a risk factor for subsequent heart attack. In fact, as we already know in this fictitious example, it is the older average age of the grey-haired group that determines their greater incidence of heart attacks. Age is a *confounder* or *confounding variable*. It confounds, or confuses, our perception of the relationship between the other two variables.

One simple definition, drawn from the standard epidemiology book, *Epidemiology in Medicine* (Hennekens and Buring, 1987), is that confounders are group differences that may affect outcome. In practice this definition means that, to be a confounder, a variable must be associated with *both* the outcome variable *and* the so-called exposure variable (the thing that you are interested in as a risk factor). In this example, age is associated *both* with having more grey hair (the exposure variable) *and* with an increasing frequency of heart attacks (the outcome variable). This is illustrated in Figure 10.1.

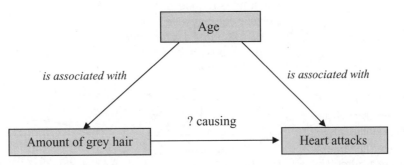

FIGURE 10.1   Representation of age confounding the causative relation between amount of grey hair and suffering a heart attack.

An observation that heart-attack victims, when compared with people without heart attacks, have an excess of grey hair is true – but it is probably a misleading explanation, with age prominent among the potential confounders.

A PLAUSIBLE EXAMPLE OF POSSIBLE CONFOUNDING

The grey hair example is an extreme scenario, divorced from real health research. Suppose instead that in a case-control study of bowel cancer (colorectal cancer) you held the hypothesis that a fibre-rich diet protected against the development of colorectal cancer. People with a diagnosis of colorectal cancer (the cases) are recruited to the study, as are some patients without cancer (the controls). All the patients in the study have their detailed dietary history taken by a dietitian. If your proposal is correct, the people in the cancer group (the cases) will have spent years eating diets that are low in fibre while the patients without cancer (the controls) have eaten rather better, with considerably higher fibre intake.

You tentatively conclude that dietary fibre protects against colorectal cancer (Figure 10.2a). But you have wondered, from the time when you were planning the study, whether smoking has anything to do with the matter. You know from your reading of published research that smoking is a fairly definite risk factor for colorectal cancer. You think it likely that people who take care to consume a diet that is high in fibre will tend to be non-smokers. Put another way, you think that 100 people whose diet is high in fibre will contain fewer smokers than will a group of 100 people who eat a low-fibre diet. Figure 10.2b shows that a researcher would be sensible to worry about the possibility that smoking is a confounder in this study because it has a likely association with both the outcome and the exposure. The next question is this: if confounding is going to be a problem in our study, what can we do about it?

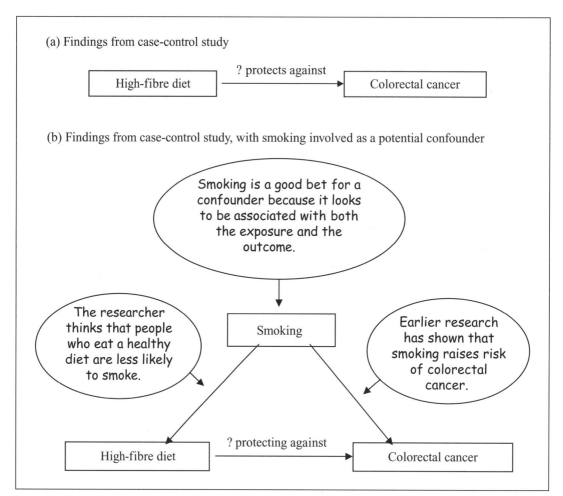

FIGURE 10.2 Representation of smoking confounding the protective relation between high fibre in the diet and colorectal cancer.

SOME WAYS TO DEAL WITH CONFOUNDING

We can use methods to deal with confounding either at the design stage of the research project, or at the data analysis stage, or both. In this chapter we are going to consider those methods which we can use at the design stage. But we will anticipate the analysis-stage methods, that are dealt with more fully in Chapter 21.

Restriction

Researchers will often apply exclusion criteria to exclude particular subjects from the study as a means of dealing with confounding. For instance, in the dietary fibre and colorectal cancer example above, we could restrict the study participants so that smokers are excluded. If we do, any connection that the study shows between poor dietary fibre and the development of colorectal cancer cannot be due to smoking – because nobody in the study smoked.

The restriction approach is straightforward and effective but as a stratagem it has at least three obvious flaws. First, it reduces the number of eligible participants; with recruitment a constant worry to researchers, we hate to use features in a study's design that keep a lot of otherwise suitable people out. Second, the findings may be regarded as applying only to the study population (non-smokers) although we want them to apply to the target population (everyone). Third, there might be an important interaction between smoking and dietary fibre and, if there is, we cannot study it if we keep out all the people who smoke.

In practice, we quite often use restriction in research but it will usually be used to trim at the edges rather than make large cuts in our sample. So, in a study of adults, we might restrict recruitment to working-age adults, because we expect an age effect and we think that there will be few older people in our sample; we would be much more reluctant to restrict the sample to males if we were to suspect an effect of gender – because it would lead perhaps to a halving of the sample. Figure 10.3 illustrates the use of restriction to tackle confounding, but where the restriction will have only a small effect on sample size and participant recruitment.

Prenatal ultrasound examinations and risk of childhood leukaemia: case-control study

Estelle Naumburg, Rino Bellocco, Sven Cnattingius, Per Hall, Anders Ekbom

To assess the impact of ultrasound and the risks of childhood lymphatic and myeloid leukaemia, we performed a nationwide population based case-control study using prospectively assembled data on prenatal exposure to ultrasound.

> The 'exposure' or risk factor under scrutiny is prenatal ultrasound examination.

Subjects, methods, and results

The cases in this study comprised all children born and diagnosed as having leukaemia between 1973 and 1989 and reported to the nationwide Swedish registers of birth, cancer, and causes of death—in all, 752 cases. One control was randomly selected for each child with leukaemia from the Swedish Birth Registry and matched by sex and year and month of birth. The study was restricted to cases and controls without Down's syndrome (n = 731), and medical records of 652 (89%) matched case-control pairs could be retrieved (578 cases with lymphatic leukaemia and 74 with myeloid leukaemia).

> Cases and controls are children with and without leukaemia.

> Children with Down syndrome are excluded, presumably because of its known link with leukaemia and a possible link with more than an average amount of prenatal ultrasound.

FIGURE 10.3   An example of restriction, used to deal with confounding in a case-control study.

Matching

Although some restriction may be useful, when it comes to dealing with potential confounders, matching is a considerably more flexible approach. Matching allows the sample to represent the whole population because it does not exclude from the study large sections of the population. For example, in a study that aimed to determine whether antidepressants were a risk factor for ischaemic heart disease (Figure 10.4) the researchers used a case-control design. Their cases and controls were people with and without heart disease, respectively. The idea was to use prescribing databases to find out whether more of those with heart disease had been prescribed antidepressants before the onset of the heart trouble. But people who do and who don't have heart disease have many differences that might confound the relation between antidepressant drugs and heart disease. Among the most obvious are age and sex. Consequently, the researchers decided to match the cases and controls for these two variables.

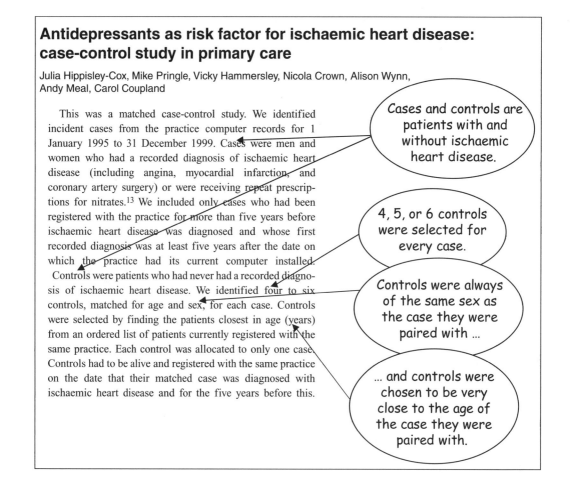

Antidepressants as risk factor for ischaemic heart disease: case-control study in primary care

Julia Hippisley-Cox, Mike Pringle, Vicky Hammersley, Nicola Crown, Alison Wynn, Andy Meal, Carol Coupland

This was a matched case-control study. We identified incident cases from the practice computer records for 1 January 1995 to 31 December 1999. Cases were men and women who had a recorded diagnosis of ischaemic heart disease (including angina, myocardial infarction, and coronary artery surgery) or were receiving repeat prescriptions for nitrates.[13] We included only cases who had been registered with the practice for more than five years before ischaemic heart disease was diagnosed and whose first recorded diagnosis was at least five years after the date on which the practice had its current computer installed. Controls were patients who had never had a recorded diagnosis of ischaemic heart disease. We identified four to six controls, matched for age and sex, for each case. Controls were selected by finding the patients closest in age (years) from an ordered list of patients currently registered with the same practice. Each control was allocated to only one case. Controls had to be alive and registered with the same practice on the date that their matched case was diagnosed with ischaemic heart disease and for the five years before this.

Cases and controls are patients with and without ischaemic heart disease.

4, 5, or 6 controls were selected for every case.

Controls were always of the same sex as the case they were paired with ...

... and controls were chosen to be very close to the age of the case they were paired with.

FIGURE 10.4   An example of matching, used to deal with confounding in a case-control study.

This method has the advantage of ensuring adequate numbers of cases and controls at each level of the confounder (at each age of patient in the above example). However, it may be difficult to find matching control subjects – especially if you are matching on more than one variable, and the method does not control for potential confounding by variables other than those that have been matched.

Statistical adjustment

This same case-control study goes on to deal with further possible confounders by adjusting for them in the statistical analysis (Figure 10.5). We deal with this kind of analysis in more detail in Chapter 21.

Antidepressants as risk factor for ischaemic heart disease: case-control study in primary care

Julia Hippisley-Cox, Mike Pringle, Vicky Hammersley, Nicola Crown, Alison Wynn, Andy Meal, Carol Coupland

Data collection

We extracted computerised data for cases and controls before the date of diagnosis (or diagnosis of matched case) using MIQUEST.[14] The data comprised name, dose, frequency, and dates of issue of all antidepressant, drugs; Read codes and dates of onset for depression, ischaemic heart disease, diabetes mellitus, and hypertension; age; sex; body mass index; most recently recorded smoking status (current smoker, former smoker, non-smoker, or not recorded); and registration date. We coded antidepressants according to the classification in the *British National Formulary* (March 2000). We determined the time (in years) between the last prescription for each antidepressant and the date of diagnosis of the case.

The researchers collected lots of information about other potential confounders ...

Statistical methods

We adjusted for the potential confounding effects of diabetes, hypertension, body mass index, and smoking status by multivariate analysis. We present the unadjusted and adjusted odds ratios associated with each dose and duration category. Dose-response relations were tested for trend. A case-control set was excluded if the information for either the case or all its controls was not known for the variable in question.

... and then used statistical models to adjust for these confounders in the analysis of the study.

FIGURE 10.5   An example of statistical modelling, to handle confounding in a case-control study.

The study chosen as an example in Figures 10.4 and 10.5 is fairly typical of case-control studies because it uses matching in the study's design for one or two variables (and age and sex are by far the commonest target variables of matching), together with statistical adjustment at the analysis stage for several other variables. The same can be said of cohort analytic studies although, for various reasons, matching is rather less common and, in consequence, adjustment is more widely used.

This book is not the place to tackle the hugely complex, technical and controversial considerations concerning matching versus statistical adjustment in research. Each has its merits and disadvantages. But it should be reasonably obvious that matching, like restriction, is a major part of the study's design. The samples are selected on the basis of any matching and restriction. Mathematical (statistical) adjustment, on the other hand, is undertaken later in the process which means, broadly speaking, that decisions over which confounders are to be dealt with can be amended as the study progresses – although any potential confounders can only be adjusted for if you have collected data about them in the first place. In Chapter 21 more will be said about the two standard methods of statistical adjustment: stratified analysis and mathematical modelling.

The use of matching, restriction, and statistical adjustment needs to be sorted out early in the planning of any study where confounding is relevant. It will need expertise, usually statistical advice.

Random allocation (randomisation)

There is a further way in which confounding can be dealt with in the design stage of clinical research: that is, in a randomised controlled trial. The trial is essentially an experiment designed to equalise confounders between the two (or occasionally more than two) experimental groups. For example, in a clinical trial of smoking cessation, patients were randomly assigned to one or other of two groups (Figure 10.6). Every

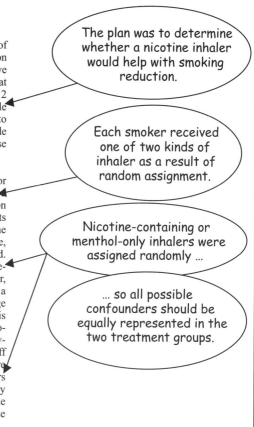

Smoking reduction with oral nicotine inhalers: double blind, randomised clinical trial of efficacy and safety

Chris T Bolliger, Jean-Pierre Zellweger, Tobias Danielsson, Xandra van Biljon, Annik Robidou, Åke Westin, André P Perruchoud, Urbain Säwe

Participants
Participants in the trial had to be at least 18 years of age, smoke 15 or more cigarettes a day, have a carbon monoxide concentration in exhaled air > 10 ppm, have smoked regularly for three or more years, have failed at least one serious attempt to quit within the past 12 months, want to reduce smoking as much as possible with the help of the nicotine inhaler, be prepared to adhere to the protocol, and be willing to provide informed consent Exclusion criteria were current use

Treatment
Independent pharmacists dispensed either active or placebo inhalers according to a computer generated randomisation list. All smokers received information about the general implications of smoking and its effects on health. Participants were asked to reduce the number of cigarettes smoked daily as much as possible, and an initial reduction of 50% was suggested.

The active treatment comprised nicotine replacement through an inhalation device (Nicorette Inhaler, Pharmacia and Upjohn).[12, 13] The inhaler consists of a plastic mouthpiece into which a disposable cartridge containing 10 mg nicotine and 1 mg menthol is inserted. At room temperature the total available nicotine content is 4-5 mg per cartridge. The inhaler delivers about 13 µg of nicotine per puff (average puff volume of 50 ml), which means that about 80 puffs are required to obtain 1 mg nicotine. The placebo inhalers were identical in appearance and contained only menthol. Both treatment groups were allowed to use the inhalers as needed, with the recommendation to use between six and 12 cartridges over 24 hours.

The plan was to determine whether a nicotine inhaler would help with smoking reduction.

Each smoker received one of two kinds of inhaler as a result of random assignment.

Nicotine-containing or menthol-only inhalers were assigned randomly …

… so all possible confounders should be equally represented in the two treatment groups.

FIGURE 10.6 An example of random allocation of treatments, used to deal with confounding in a randomised controlled trial of nicotine inhalers for smoking reduction.

patient received an inhaler but while one group's inhaler contained only menthol, the other delivered menthol with nicotine. The experiment thereby aimed to determine whether an oral nicotine inhaler can result in sustained reduction in smoking.

In a randomised controlled trial the allocation to two groups by the play of chance means that, theoretically at least, both groups should have the same characteristics until the treatment begins. This process means (in the above nicotine study, for example) that there ought to be a similar profile in both treatment groups of any confounders – such as age, sex, current smoking habits, nicotine dependence, psychological characteristics that might influence ability to stop smoking, and so on. In fact, there may well be confounders whose effects are completely unknown to the researcher. But whether a confounder is known or unknown, measurable or not, random allocation should distribute it equally between the two treatment groups.

Unfortunately, in practice this option is only available when we are dealing with trials of treatment. Looking back at the earlier examples in this chapter, we can't randomly assign people to long-term antidepressant drugs to see whether they get a rise in heart-attack rates; much less can we subject unborn children to ultrasound examinations to examine leukaemia rates. Because random allocation only applies to treatment trials, early career researchers designing their own study will usually be dealing with confounding in non-experimental research – using restriction, matching, and statistical adjustment.

Dinesh

As the plan for his study evolves it seems clear that Dinesh is going to investigate a single sample of patients who have self-harmed, determining some of their group characteristics and following them up to estimate repetition rates. The analysis of these data will provide information that will be of value for the planning of a randomised controlled trial that may or may not be undertaken later. He will not need therefore, to deal with confounding because he will not be trying to compare outcomes between groups.

He will, however, be establishing whether characteristics such as sex, age, method of self-harm (overdose of medicines or self-cutting, for example), and history of previous self-harm, are related to repetition rate. If any of these variables does have a clear association with repetition of self-harm then this information will be valuable for the planning of a later trial. We don't tackle the matter here, but random allocation in trials often involves stratified random allocation and Dinesh's work will help to determine which variables should be considered for such stratification; a useful short article about how to randomise is Altman and Bland's *BMJ* article (1999).

One final word of caution: it is really important to deal with confounders but the more measures you take in an effort to do so, the more complex (and usually larger) your study will become. If in your first project you are making comparisons and will need to consider confounding, we suggest that you concentrate on those factors that will make your results uninterpretable if you don't deal with them, and leave more speculative confounders for further work. This nearly always means dealing at least with gender and age. Any other potentially major confounders should be reasonably obvious and will vary according to the study in question.

11

How Many People to Study?

SAMPLE SIZE

Now is about the time for you to decide how many subjects you will need for your investigation – how big a sample. The approaches (and the underlying philosophy) to this question differ between qualitative and quantitative research, so we'll treat them separately and begin with the quantitative case.

GETTING THE APPROPRIATE SAMPLE SIZE IF YOUR RESEARCH IS QUANTITATIVE

As far as sample size is concerned, you want to recruit as few people as is necessary because:

- it's easier, cheaper, and less time-consuming, and . . .
- it's more ethical.

However, you must have enough subjects to ensure that if there is anything going on, you'll find it.

The essential concept here is *power*. The power of a statistical procedure is its ability to detect an effect if there is one present. It's a bit like using a magnifying glass – the stronger the magnification the more likely you are to detect something really small. Suppose we use statistical procedures which have 80% power. This means that there is an 80% chance that if there's something to find, you will find it. Power and sample size are linked – the bigger the sample size, the greater the power. So how big a sample size will you need to get 80% power?

This is probably a good time for you to do a bit of reading on the meaning of statistical power, sample size, and their calculation. You should also, if you have access to a medical statistician, go and talk to her or him about your sample size question (besides, if you're doing quantitative research it's always a good idea to be on good terms with a statistician). You will also get quite a few hits if you type 'power calculation' or 'sample size calculation' into Google. Alternatively, there are a number of web sites that you can use. For example, http://www.stat.uiowa.edu/~rlenth/Power/.

Calculating the appropriate sample size is a three-step process as shown below. You will have to:

- Decide on the power level you want – 80% or 90% is usual;
- Decide on a confidence level – usually 95%; or a level of significance – a value of 0.05 is usual (we explain what these terms mean below);
- Decide on the minimum clinically useful size of the effect (or change, or difference, etc.) that you want to be able to detect.

Getting Started in Health Research, First Edition. David Bowers, Allan House and David Owens.
© 2011 David Bowers, Allan House and David Owens. Published 2011 by Blackwell Publishing Ltd.

A confidence level refers to the degree of confidence that you place in your estimate (your intelligent guess) of a value which you are estimating. This is expressed as a confidence interval (CI). For example, suppose, in a trial of a growth hormone for the treatment of children of restricted growth, the researchers estimate from their sample data that the mean difference in the growth in height over a one-year period, between a group of children given the growth hormone and a group of children given a placebo, is 1.25cm, with a 95% level of confidence of (0.98 to 1.52)cm. In other words they are saying that they are 95% confident that the true mean difference in growth is between 0.98cm and 1.52cm.

The level of statistical significance (also known as the alpha, or α level) is the probability of getting a false positive, that is, you think that you've found an effect (a difference in mean height in this example) when there actually isn't one. The smaller alpha is, the smaller is this risk. We will consider it in more detail in Part VI of this book, but a value of 0.05 is pretty much standard in clinical research.

You need to decide on the minimum size of the effect that you think is clinically interesting. This means that, for example, if you are investigating a new drug for hypertension, you probably won't be much interested in a reduction in mean diastolic blood pressure of 1mmHg in your treatment group, but you might think that 10mmHg would be worthwhile.

As an example of power and sample size, researchers who were investigating whether chloramphenicol, or a combination of benzylpenicillin and gentamicin, would be better for the treatment of severe pneumonia in children in Papua New Guinea, were interested in comparing adverse outcomes as well as mortality, between the two drug regimens. A description of their sample size deliberation is shown in Figure 11.1.

Chloramphenicol versus benzylpenicillin and gentamicin for the treatment of severe pneumonia in children in Papua New Guinea: a randomised trial

Trevor Duke, Harry Poka, Frank Dale, Audrey Michael, Joyce Mgone, Tilda Wal

A minimum sample size of n=1154 is required to ...

... detect a difference of 30% in the per cent of children with adverse outcomes when ...

... power is set at 80%, and α at 0.05 ...

In a sample of 100 children with severe pneumonia treated with chloramphenicol in the year before the study began there was a total adverse outcome of 22%. A sample size of 1154 patients was based on testing for a 30% difference in adverse outcome between the two antibiotic regimens, with 80% power, and an alpha level of 0.05 (two-sided test of proportions). A sample size of 1114 would test whether there was a 40% difference in mortality between the two regimens (80% power and an alpha level of 0.05).

... whereas to detect a difference of 40% in mortality requires a sample size of 1114.

FIGURE 11.1   An example of power in a sample size calculation from a study of treatments for severe pneumonia in children.

Dinesh

You will remember that Dinesh originally planned to do a trial comparing the proportion of subjects re-attending within six months (his outcome measure) among those using an advocacy service and those not. However, he was persuaded that this was too ambitious a project to do in the time he had available and in the light of his inexperience as a researcher. Instead he is going to explore the practicalities and problems associated with doing such a trial in the future. For example, whether there is a big enough throughput of patients in his hospital, the proportion re-attending within six months, the proportion who might agree to accept the help of an advocate, ethical issues, measures of patient satisfaction and mood, practical issues related to access to patients (where and when to recruit), patient selection, administrative and clinical staff co-operation, and so on.

Patient throughput, re-attendance patterns (a colleague tells him that the current six-month figure is around 16%), and drop-out rates, he can get retrospectively from patient records. Issues around patient access and staff co-operation he can tackle by talking to management and sounding out the clinical staff likely to be involved. But he is going to have to do a small-ish prospective study to choose and to road-test suitable patient mood and satisfaction scales, and to determine patient attitudes to using an advocate. Dinesh understands that one of the things that will be needed if a trial proper is to go ahead is a calculation of the sample size needed to provide reasonably narrow confidence intervals for his measurements of mood and of satisfaction. He decides to consult a statistician for advice on how to do this.

GETTING THE APPROPRIATE SAMPLE SIZE IF YOUR RESEARCH IS QUALITATIVE

In qualitative research you select your sample according to certain key criteria. This is to ensure that all those key groups in the population who can throw light on your research question are included in your sample. Moreover, you need to have enough diversity within each of the key criteria to enable you to explore fully any differences in attitudes and behaviours.

For example, age and sex are often key selection criteria. If you were exploring the attitudes and beliefs of men and women to abortion, you might believe that these attitudes vary according to both age and sex. In this case you would want to ensure that you could investigate this thoroughly by making sure that you had enough age bands for both the men and the women in your sample.

With qualitative research your sample will usually be considerably smaller than is typical in quantitative research. There are four reasons for this:

- First, as a qualitative researcher, you will usually work with information-rich subjects hoping that each one of them will provide a lot of information.
- Second, unlike in a quantitative research project, you are not trying to measure prevalence, for example what percentage of men are opposed to abortion, but only the attitudes of men (even one man) to abortion.
- Third, the data collection methods you are most likely to use, principally the face-to-face interview, is both time- and resource-consuming. (We will discuss data collection in more detail in Chapter 18.) Moreover, you will subsequently need to transcribe the recording (or write out detailed notes if you prefer note taking) afterwards. Each of these has then to be analysed. The analysis even of a single interview can take a long time. (We will consider the analysis of qualitative data in Chapter 18.)
- Fourth, you will reach a point where the analysis of each additional interview produces little in the way of new information – this is known as the saturation or data redundancy point.

In Chapter 8 you had to decide on the type of sample most appropriate to the aim or purpose of your study, for example an extreme-case sample, a typical-case sample, a maximum-variation or heterogeneous sample, and so on. We saw that Anna decided to use a maximum-variation sample. But how big a sample will she (and will you) need? There are virtually no guidelines for determining sample size in qualitative research, but two crucial factors need to be considered: the number of selection criteria; and the degree of diversity within each of them. Inevitably, the larger both of these are, the larger will be your sample. A population with little diversity would be labelled as homogeneous. In this case, you would not need as large a sample to get reasonable coverage. Now let's get back to Anna.

Anna

Anna has decided to recruit a maximum variation (or maximum diversity or heterogeneous) sample. After she has done some reading, talked with colleagues, and drawn from her own experience with mothers, Anna jots down what she believes are most likely to be her key selection criteria (there are five of these – see Figure 11.2).

The 'jab status' of mothers √

Mother's age √

Education level of mother √

Household income √

Baby's number of older siblings √

FIGURE 11.2   Anna lists the characteristics (the criteria) she needs to consider when she chooses her sample.

Her approach is straightforward. She will use the centre's medical records to identify and allocate mothers to each of the three 'jab' groups – mothers who: have brought their babies for the MMR jab (group 1); have asked for single jabs (group 2); have done neither of these (group 3). She will then start to interview them, choosing one from each group in turn. She has already decided to use a semi-structured interview with a topic guide (see Chapter 9), and to record each interview. (We will have more to say about collecting and recording data in Chapter 18.) Before she gets into the attitudes and beliefs part of each interview, she will confirm the subject's age, and then ask about education, income, and baby's older siblings. If from these answers she finds that she already has enough mothers in any particular category she won't go on with the rest of the interview.

(Anna also has in mind a couple of possible additional criteria – ethnicity, for one – but she feels that these can be left out for now – she knows that the larger the number of criteria, the larger the potential sample size.)

She now chooses some *categories* to enable each of her five criteria to be fully explored. For the age criterion, for example, she is unsure how age will be related to attitudes, so she decide on two age categories – less than 25, or 25 or more. (If she felt that greater sensitivity is needed for younger mothers, then her categories might have been: 16–24, 25–34, 35 or more; but the fewer the categories the better in terms of limiting sample size.) Trying to keep things as simple as possible for now, Anna chooses the categories shown in Figure 11.3 – giving her 11 categories in total. She thinks she could aim to get two mothers in each category to start with, which means a sample size of 22.

After a small number of interviews Anna will transcribe and analyse each one (see Chapter 22 for a discussion on the analysis of interview material), trying to identify themes and the sort of information that is emerging. This may cause her to amend the structure of her interview. She will continue with this procedure until no new themes seem to be appearing – this point is called saturation or data redundancy.

```
┌─────────────────────────────────────────────────────────────┐
│  The 'jab status' of mothers        1, 2, 3                  │
│                                                             │
│  Mother's age                       < 25; ≥ 25              │
│                                                             │
│  Cessation of FT education          ≤ 16; > 16             │
│                                                             │
│  Household income £p.a.             < £30k; ≥ £30k         │
│                                                             │
│  Baby's number of older siblings  0; ≥ 1                   │
└─────────────────────────────────────────────────────────────┘
```

FIGURE 11.3   Anna specifies the categories to be represented in her sample.

The sample selection criteria matrix

Anna could have used (and you may want to) a somewhat more structured approach to select her sample, by using a sample selection matrix, as shown in Figure 11.4. The number of subjects shown here in each cell is known as the quota. The quotas specify the number of subjects that will be needed with each of the characteristics set out in the matrix. It is usual to specify the quotas as a range, as here, rather than as an exact number. Notice that Anna has chosen to have the cessation of full-time education criterion defined solely by age. In other words, among the approximately 8 mothers aged less than 25 years, she hopes to recruit about 3–5 who will have ceased full-time education by 16, and another 3–5 after 16. Note that there will be three of these matrices – one for each of the jab status groups.

	Less than 25y		25y or more	
	Less than £30k	£30k or more	Less than £30k	£30k or more
No. older siblings = 0	1–2	1–2	1–2	1–2
No. older siblings = 1 or more	1–2	1–2	1–2	1–2
	Education across age groups			
FT education up to 16	3–5		3–5	
FT education 16+	3–5		3–5	

FIGURE 11.4   An example of a sample selection matrix, with quotas, based on Anna's project.

A WORD OF WARNING ON SATURATION

Exactly when the saturation point is arrived at will rely a lot on your judgement and experience, but you need to be careful not to stop the data collection prematurely. This may happen if you:

- Have a sample which is too narrowly defined – that is, lacking some important criteria;
- The sample you have selected is not information-rich enough;
- Your interview or analysis skills are not enabling you to 'get through' to the core feelings, beliefs, attitudes or behaviours, of your subjects; and so you have not been able to identify some important themes.

As an example, suppose you were investigating ways of influencing pregnant women to stop smoking during pregnancy. You might have face-to-face interviews with a group of such women and find, surprisingly, that you get saturation after seeing only eight of them. But this may be because your group doesn't include any women who have had higher education, or who have a partner who smokes, or who are aged over 35, and so on. The addition of some appropriate extra criteria may well have thrown up new themes.

An illustration of how few subjects may be needed before the saturation point is reached comes from a study on care-seeking among women with postpartum depression, where the authors reported that, 'A total of 18 women participated in the study as data redundancy was achieved with this sample.'

WHAT YOU NEED TO DO NOW – A CHECK LIST

- Decide on your key selection criteria.
- Decide on the categories within each criterion. This will depend on how much diversity you think that there might be in each criterion. There should be enough categories to allow each criterion to be fully explored.
- Decide on the number of subjects you think will suffice in each category.

You can change any of these factors later in the light of your data-collecting experience. In the next chapter we look at the sort of preparations you need to make in readiness for your analysis.

12

Getting Ready for a Qualitative Analysis

BE PREPARED

In Chapter 18 we will discuss the actual collection of your research data, and in Chapters 21 and 22 we will examine the various approaches to its analysis. However, before you can either collect or subsequently analyse your data, there are a number of things that you must plan for. The following is a check list of the most important of them.

- If you are planning to interview individuals for your research, have you decided where you are going to do this? Will it be in a subject's home, workplace, or elsewhere? Have you sorted this out, and made sure that the location you have decided upon is suitable – that you will be free from interruption, that the room will be secure and comfortable, will be spacious enough, and so on. Will you need to provide water, or other refreshment? Have you made arrangements for this? If you or somebody else will be spending time alone with the person you are interviewing, will you be safe? (see Chapter 18).
- How long will each interview take? How many can you fit into your schedule? You are probably going to need at least an hour for each one. You will also need time between interviews to take stock, make notes, rest, and so on. Two interviews in a morning and/or afternoon is probably all you will be able to manage. If you are travelling to and from the interview location (e.g. a subject's home) you will need to allow time for this. So before you start you will need to block out enough time in your calendar for the number of interviews you have decided upon – 10? 15?
- If you intend to use a topic guide you must make sure that you are totally familiar with it, so that you need to refer to it as little as possible during the interview – if at all. Bear in mind that you might need to tweak the guide after the first one or two interviews.
- Will all of your subjects have a good command of English? If there are any who do not, you will need to organise a translator to sit in with you and interpret your questions and the subject's responses. In some situations you might want to consider matching the gender of the interviewer with the subject.
- Recording interviews is believed by some researchers to be better than note taking, although there is no reason why you shouldn't make a few notes during an interview and as many as you want shortly afterwards. Make sure you are familiar with the recording equipment and how best to use it. It's essential to have a dummy run with a volunteer colleague. And remember to check the recording after each interview.
- Interviews will almost certainly need to be transcribed. Who will do this? If not you, then who? If someone is going to help you, have you made an arrangement for this? Will they need to be paid?
- If any recorded interviews will be in a foreign language, have you got a translator lined up?

Getting Started in Health Research, First Edition. David Bowers, Allan House and David Owens.
© 2011 David Bowers, Allan House and David Owens. Published 2011 by Blackwell Publishing Ltd.

- Are you likely to make video recordings? Make sure you can use the video recorder (checking sound levels and lighting, for example). Again do a dummy run. How are you going to transfer the information therein? What about photographic data? Consider storage and security issues with this sort of material.

- How do you intend to deal with any documents given to you by the patient, for example letters, notes, photos, and so on. Do you have a proper system for filing and storing these?

- What methods will you use to analyse your data? There are a variety of methods which you can use depending on the nature of your enquiry, the type of data you have collected, the theoretical underpinnings of your research philosophy (grounded theory versus content analysis versus narrative analysis, and so on). If you are not already familiar with these analytic concepts then you will need to do a fair amount of reading beforehand (and discuss any questions with your supervisor).

- Are you going to analyse your data 'by hand'? If not, have you identified and made yourself familiar with any software appropriate for such an analysis? For example, NVivo 7, or ATLAS.ti. A tutorial in the use of NVivo 7 is available via: http://www.sagepub.co.uk/richards/. Other useful sources for analytic software are described in: http://www.content-analysis.de/software/qualitative-analysis and http://www.eval.org/resources/listservs.asp.

Anna

Anna has decided to interview mothers in her consulting room at the practice, although she is prepared to do home visits if this is really necessary. She obviously knows her room well and feels comfortable there. Most of the mothers (if not all) have been to it on at least a few occasions before, so should find the surroundings reasonably familiar, secure, and hopefully relaxing. The room is certainly big enough.

She plans to record each interview using her digital voice recorder, which she has used in the past and is very familiar with. All of the patients on her list of potential participants speak and understand English, so she won't need a translator.

She has written a topic guide and is familiar with it.

She has one half-day a week free which she plans to use to do her interviewing. She reckons that each interview will last about an hour, or possibly a little longer. She hopes to fit at least one and possibly two interviews into each session.

One of the reception staff is a good typist and has offered to transcribe the recordings for her, and store them electronically (in MS Word probably). There is enough money in the budget to pay her for this.

Anna needs to decide on a method of analysis. She is acutely aware that she is a novice researcher, and that qualitative research is a complex and potentially difficult subject area, so she has decided not to be too ambitious and to keep things as simple as possible – this being her first effort. In terms of her analytic approach she decides to use content analysis. This will mean identifying key themes, categories, and concepts from the transcripts. For now she is undecided whether to analyse her data by hand or use one of the existing computer-assisted qualitative data analysis packages – she's heard that NVivo might be suitable and not too difficult to use. She knows that she will need to do quite a lot of reading on the identification of themes and concepts, and so on, before she gets to the analysis stage.

Moreover, Anna will need to think about data management. Her raw data will be a series of transcripts, unorganised and uninformative. How to proceed? The first stage will be to sort it in some relevant and helpful way, so she needs to make some decisions about this – maybe by age or educational level of mother, for example. She might then want to read through a few of the transcripts to get some idea of what she's got – how diverse are the responses, how lengthy (or not), how clear or confused, and so on. This initial familiarisation with the raw material might start to throw up some initial themes and ideas.

In conjunction with these thoughts, Anna will want to consider how she can store her data so that its confidentiality is assured.

Once she feels that she is reasonably familiar with the material, she will go through the transcripts one by one and try to identify important themes and ideas present in each. She knows that she is likely to end up with a long list of these. She will then need to study this list to see if there are links between any of the themes. These can then be grouped together into a series of main themes or categories, each of which will contain a number of subthemes. This arrangement of main themes and subthemes is often known as the index.

When Anna is satisfied that her list – her index – is reasonably comprehensive (it's not set in stone, she can re-visit it at any time) she can then apply it to the raw data, going through each transcript, reading every word, phrase, and sentence very carefully, deciding what it is about, what it means, and then labelling it, and then allocating each to the appropriate part, or parts, of the index. The final step will be for Anna to attempt to synthesise and summarise her data.

She has heard of the concept of framework analysis and its use for the data management problem, and decides to read up on this before she goes any further. She knows that once a (smallish) number of main themes have been identified (each with its associated subthemes), each main theme can then be charted into its own matrix. Every respondent is allocated a row, with the columns corresponding to subthemes. She understands that a spreadsheet program can be easily adopted for this. She is going to have to find out something about spreadsheets, and hopes that the practice manager can help out, but she has yet to make a firm decision about whether to use this approach.

Once Anna has done all this preliminary work she will be ready to start her study.

13

Getting Ready for a Quantitative Analysis

GETTING READY

In Chapter 12 we looked at the preparations you will need to make prior to analysing the data that you have collected if your research project is qualitative. In this chapter we are going to discuss the same sorts of things but for the *quantitative* research case. Here you will have to prepare to deal with the following issues:

- Where are you going to store your data before you start your analysis? On paper? Using MS Word? Or MS Excel? (This question is dealt with more fully in Chapters 18 and 19.)
- You will need to produce a table of basic characteristics, which will describe the principal features of your subjects. Which characteristics are you going to enquire about or collect? Which ones are relevant?
- You will almost certainly need to provide some descriptive statistics to go with this basic table (proportions, means/medians, interquartile ranges, standard deviations, and so on). Which ones?
- What method of analysis will you use? For example, are you doing no more than calculating prevalences? Will you be comparing two means, or two proportions? Will you want to calculate odds ratios, or risk ratios, and so on. We discuss a few of the possibilities below.
- How are you going to present all of these items? With tables and/or charts, with text? Which combination will work best?
- How are you going to take into account any potential confounders (Chapter 10)?
- Are you sure that you know how to do all of these things – or at least know someone who can provide some help?

WHICH METHOD OF ANALYSIS?

Each piece of research will require its own appropriate analytic approach (and this will depend on the research question and the chosen research design). Unfortunately, there are so many different types of statistical analyses available (some quite simple, some much more complex) that we cannot describe any of them in any detail here. If you are not completely confident about these methods, you can get some guidance from your supervisor, but you will almost certainly benefit from consulting your friendly medical statistician. In any case you should have access to a good medical statistics book, for example Altman

(1995), Bowers *et al.* (2006), or Bowers (2008). However, here is a list of the most common approaches which you might find helpful.

- *To determine prevalence (simple cross-sectional design, one or more groups).*
  Here a simple percentage(s) or proportion(s) will do the job.
- *To compare proportions in two or more independent groups (are they the same?).*
  Use a chi-squared test, or calculate a confidence interval for the difference in proportions, or a risk ratio and its confidence interval.
- *To compare two means (are they the same?).*
  With independent groups (and metric Normally distributed data) calculate confidence intervals based on the 2-sample t-test (a parametric procedure). With matched groups calculate confidence intervals based on the 1-sample t-test.
- *To compare two medians (are they the same?).*
  With independent groups (and ordinal or non-Normal metric data) use the Mann-Whitney test. With matched groups (and with ordinal or non-Normal metric data) use the Wilcoxon test. These are non-parametric procedures.
- *To determine if two variables are independent.*
  Use the chi-squared test or simple regression.
- *To determine risk and odds ratios (and numbers needed to treat).*
  Use simple contingency table analysis for unadjusted ratios; to control for confounders use stratified contingency tables (or logistic regression – see next paragraph).
- *To examine the relationship between variables (and identify risk factors).*
  With a metric outcome variable use linear regression; with a binary outcome variable use logistic regression (in both cases adjust for confounders).
- *To determine if two variables agree.*
  Use Bland-Altman for metric data, kappa for categorical data.
- *To see if two variables are associated.*
  Use correlation analysis.
- *To examine the qualities of a diagnostic test procedure.*
  Calculate sensitivity, specificity, likelihood ratios (possibly), and ROC curves.
- *To compare survival in two or more groups.*
  Use Kaplan-Meier survival analysis and the log-rank test. To control for confounders use Cox regression and calculate hazard ratios.

You will also need to decide beforehand on a level of significance before you examine the statistical significance of your results (see Chapter 11, 0.05 is usual). You should be familiar with the appropriate use of p-values and confidence intervals.

In addition to choosing an appropriate method of analysis, you will also need to be able to apply it using some suitable statistics program. SPSS is perhaps the most readily available in the health service, but Minitab and Stata are also suitable possibilities. You will have to make sure you have ready access to one of these packages, and know either how to do the analysis you have decided on yourself, or have someone you can consult to help you out.

You need to prepare for these matters before you go any further. One useful way to start is to prepare your results tables before you have any data. Now let's see what Dinesh is up to.

Dinesh

You will recall that Dinesh's original idea was to do a clinical trial on the efficacy of an advocacy service for self-harm patients in reducing the average time to re-attendance (his main outcome variable). He will also want to measure patient mood and satisfaction. However, he was advised that a clinical trial would take too long – considerably longer than the time he has available – and would require more expertise than he has acquired so far. Instead he decided to identify the potential problems and feasibility issues (practical and clinical) with the idea that sometime in the future he may be able to do a clinical trial. These might include things like: Will there be enough patients passing through the ED in a reasonable time scale – enough to meet his sample size calculation at least? (see Chapter 11). Will enough people consent? What proportion are likely to drop out? Will clinical staff be willing to co-operate? What will clinical management think? What are the ethical issues? Where will the advocates come from? Will patients agree to use an advocate? And so on.

Dinesh makes a list of his questions (see Figure 13.1).

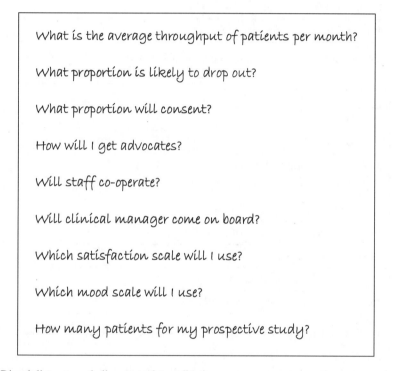

What is the average throughput of patients per month?

What proportion is likely to drop out?

What proportion will consent?

How will I get advocates?

Will staff co-operate?

Will clinical manager come on board?

Which satisfaction scale will I use?

Which mood scale will I use?

How many patients for my prospective study?

FIGURE 13.1   Dinesh lists some challenges to data collection.

He can get the answers to some of these problems (patient throughput, drop-out rate, time to re-attend, etc.) retrospectively from the department's case records, but to measure things like the proportion willing to consent to using an advocate, and for measurement of mood and satisfaction, he proposes to do a small-scale prospective descriptive study to establish some parameters (for which he will need ethical consent). Dinesh has already decided to obtain these data from a face-to-face interview in the respondent's home. In Chapter 9 he was undecided on both a mood and a satisfaction measure, but he does know that it is better to use an existing scale wherever possible. As part of his preparations he now needs to decide which scales he will use and then familiarise himself with them, their administration, and their scoring and interpretation. After taking advice he decides to use the PHQ9 scale to measure mood and a simple Likert scale for satisfaction.

Dinesh knows that he will need to summarise the basic characteristics of patients whose data he gets from clinical records, as well as those from his prospective or follow-up study. He envisages baseline tables similar to those in Figures 13.2 and 13.3.

	n=
Male (no. %)	
Age (mean & s.d.)	

Method of self-harm (index episode)
    Cutting (no. %)
    Poisoning (no. %)
    Other (no. %)	

With previous history of self-harm (no. %)	
Dropped out (no. %)	
Time to re-attendance (median; IQR)	

FIGURE 13.2   Dinesh's draft baseline table for patient data from clinical records.

	n=
Male (no. %)	
Age (mean & s.d.)	

Method of self-harm (index episode)
    Cutting (no. %)
    Poisoning (no. %)
    Other (no. %)	

With previous history of self-harm (no. %)	
Willing to use an advocate (no. %)	
Mood score (median; interquartile range)	
Satisfaction score (median; interquartile range	

FIGURE 13.3   Dinesh's draft baseline table for patient data from follow-up or prospective study.

In Chapter 3 you wrote down your initial plan. In the next chapter you will see how to set out your final protocol. You will use this as a guide – a sort of road map – to what you are doing and where you are going. It is also essential for obtaining ethical consent (see Chapter 16).

14

Writing Your Final Protocol

You should now be in a position to write out a final protocol for your study. Protocols vary greatly in length – up to many dozens of pages perhaps for a multi-centre international trial of a new drug. But we are thinking here of something much shorter – about two sides of A4.

This protocol will be useful in a number of ways:

- You can send it to people whom you want to consult as a convenient summary of what you are up to;
- It provides a summary that can be appended to other official documents – for example an application for approval from a research ethics committee (see Chapter 16) or to register for PhD studies;
- You can use it as a framework for writing up your research project when it is eventually completed.

Figure 14.1 summarises the structure and contents of a typical research protocol.

- Background
- Aims and hypotheses
- Methods
  - design
  - setting
  - sample
  - measures
  - analysis
- Feasibility
- Ethical considerations
- Support

FIGURE 14.1   Components of a research protocol.

Here is a reminder of what each section should contain.

Getting Started in Health Research, First Edition. David Bowers, Allan House and David Owens.

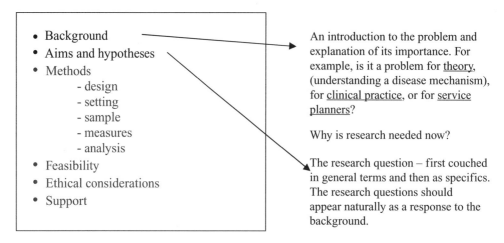

- Background
- Aims and hypotheses
- Methods
    - design
    - setting
    - sample
    - measures
    - analysis
- Feasibility
- Ethical considerations
- Support

An introduction to the problem and explanation of its importance. For example, is it a problem for <u>theory</u>, (understanding a disease mechanism), for <u>clinical practice</u>, or for <u>service planners</u>?

Why is research needed now?

The research question – first couched in general terms and then as specifics. The research questions should appear naturally as a response to the background.

FIGURE 14.2   Start your protocol with a clear statement of the problem you want to address.

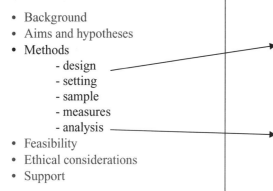

- Background
- Aims and hypotheses
- Methods
    - design
    - setting
    - sample
    - measures
    - analysis
- Feasibility
- Ethical considerations
- Support

With the help of an experienced adviser it should be possible to describe your research methods well. The acid test is whether they will lead to results that answer the research question!

It is surprising how often researchers start data collection without a properly worked up <u>analysis plan</u> – quantitative or qualitative.

FIGURE 14.3   Outline your research design.

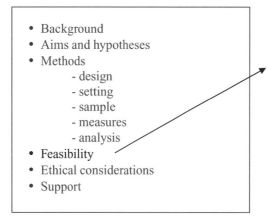

- Background
- Aims and hypotheses
- Methods
    - design
    - setting
    - sample
    - measures
    - analysis
- Feasibility
- Ethical considerations
- Support

Some questions to cover explicitly in your protocol:

- how will I identify, approach and recruit participants?
- will I be able to recruit enough participants in the time I have?
- does the setting of my research pose particular problems (working in prisons, out of hours, lots of travel)
- do I need the co-operation of others, such as busy clinicians, and how will I get it?
- will I (or anybody else) need training to do the research?
- have I identified all the costs?

FIGURE 14.4   Consider practical aspects of doing the research.

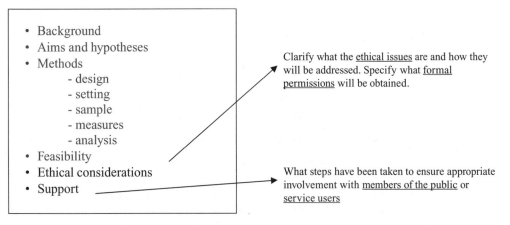

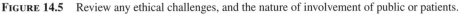

FIGURE 14.5   Review any ethical challenges, and the nature of involvement of public or patients.

Dinesh and Anna both need to come up with a research protocol. The annex at the end of this chapter contains their ideas.

In the next chapter we turn to the need faced by many researchers – the need to obtain funding – obviously much more important for large-scale projects.

ANNEX   DINESH'S AND ANNA'S RESEARCH PROTOCOLS

Dinesh's protocol

Background

Most people who harm themselves deliberately and seek medical help present to the emergency department. They describe unpleasant experiences there and there are high rates of departure before assessment and treatment is complete. Similarly, ED staff reports suggest high rates of dissatisfaction. Return rates are high and improving the experience of service may be a means to achieving improvement in outcomes. A plausible intervention is delivery of an advocacy service, to be evaluated in an RCT, but before such a study is undertaken we need to know a number of things:

(1) What are the rates of attendance, early departure rates and six-month reattendance rates for adults who come to ED after self-harm?
(2) What are current rates of satisfaction with services, and mood disorder, in attenders?
(3) What proportion of patients attending will consent to a research assessment and will complete measures, and what proportion express interest in an advocacy service if one were available?

Study design: Prospective cohort study

Setting: The Emergency Department of Celesteville General Hospital

Sample: All adults (>18 years) presenting to the ED after an episode of self-poisoning or self-injury

Exclusions: unable to consent, for example, due to intoxication, conscious level, delirium, learning disability

Measures: Demographic: age, gender, ethnicity, language spoken

Self-harm: nature of act
conscious level
intoxication
outcome of episode in ED
time to reattendance for self-harm (up to six months)

Mood: PHQ9

Satisfaction with services: (Likert scale)

Interest in advocacy services if available (Likert scale).

Demographic data and details of the self-harm will be collected using a standardised proforma attached to the ED chart at booking-in, and checked later against clinical record and ED database. Mood scale and satisfaction scale will be handed to patients as they leave ED and completed during the next week.

Analysis plan:

(a) Simple descriptive statistics – number and percentages for all variables
– means/medians for mood and satisfaction
(b) Multivariate – two models with global satisfaction and with repetition as dependent variables. The former will be a regression model and the latter will be either a regression model (repetition at six months) or survival analysis.

Feasibility: To start in spring to avoid staff pressures due to winter surge in infections and accidents.

Ethics: Written information will need to be very brief and simple given circumstances, and we will seek either signed or witnessed verbal consent. We will obtain LREC approval. Individual patient identifiers are needed to allow follow-up to six months reattendance rates. Once those results are obtained then all individual identifiers will be replaced by unique study identifiers. Research reports and manuscripts for publication will contain no material that will allow identification of individual participants. The local research ethics committee will be approached for approval to undertake the study.

Anna's protocol

Background
A published case series proposing a possible association between MMR vaccination and later onset of childhood autism led to widespread public concern about the safety of the vaccination, and a substantial drop in vaccination rates. Despite the robust epidemiological evidence to the contrary, and the discrediting of the original work, rates of take-up of childhood MMR vaccination have not returned to acceptable levels and we do not fully understand why.

Study design: Cross-sectional observational study
Setting: Greendale Health Centre (Primary Care)
Sample: Mothers of children eligible for MMR. Quota sampling:
– mothers whose children have been given MMR
– mothers seeking separate administration of vaccines
– mother declining/not attending for vaccination

Exclusions: – unable to give consent
  – known contra-indication to MMR
  – mothers of children under statutory provision (e.g. care order)

Method: Semi-structured one-to-one interview based on topic guide.
  Main themes to cover:
  – experience and knowledge about vaccination
  – knowledge of MMR controversy
  – current views on vaccination: risks + benefits
  – sources of advice

Analysis plan: Interviews will be recorded and transcribed. A thematic framework analysis will be conducted on the transcripts.

Feasibility: The principal researcher will approach all women for consent and undertake all interviews. A review of GP register indicates that there are 311 eligible mothers currently in the practice.

Ethics: Mothers will give written consent following explanation and receipt of an information sheet. Tapes and transcripts will be anonymised and stored in a secure place separately from clinical records. They will not be made available to other practice staff. Research reports and manuscripts for publication will contain no material that will allow identification of individual participants. The local research ethics committee will be approached for approval to undertake the study.

15

Arranging Funding

DECIDING WHAT FUNDING IS REQUIRED

The first step towards raising the money to pay for your project – applying for a research grant – is to work out what money you will need. You have a number of things (at least five) to decide. For a start, is any payment for equipment or materials required? Second, are there any services that you will have to pay for? Third, who is undertaking the work, and will that person (or persons) be receiving a salary for working on the project? For a first project you, and perhaps a willing colleague or two, may expect to do the work in your available time, so there will be no extra salaries to be paid; for subsequent and bigger projects the field work will usually be undertaken by designated and employed research staff – often taken on specifically for that purpose. Fourth, will there be transport costs for anyone involved with the project? Fifth, will you be paying fees for publishing or otherwise disseminating your findings?

Costs:	Examples:
Equipment or materials	Computer, printer, paper, software, printed data sheets, postage stamps, recording equipment (for interviews), new cyclotron . . .
Services	Training (in a technique perhaps), transcribing recorded interviews, telephone calls, video conferencing, data entry on to computers, optical scanning of data sheets, health service activity (such as case record retrieval), blood or urine tests, fees for tracing of death records (perhaps from national statistics offices), statistical support . . .
Salaries	Research assistant, therapists, data manager, your own time (your employer might require financial compensation for your time) . . .
Transport	Researchers' travel (to training, or research conference, or to participants' homes . . .); participants' travel (to and from hospital) . . .
Publishing	Payment to on-line journals for publication of research papers, publishing a monograph or report . . . .

You can see, just from these examples, that there is an enormous range of potential costs in running a project. Of course it is fairly easy to work out the costs in a small project but it may still need financial support along these lines – even if only in a modest way.

Getting Started in Health Research, First Edition. David Bowers, Allan House and David Owens.
© 2011 David Bowers, Allan House and David Owens. Published 2011 by Blackwell Publishing Ltd.

Equipment and materials

Equipment and materials costs are usually fairly straightforward to estimate. Purchase costs are easy to determine, and it is often reasonably simple to estimate how many letters you plan to send out or how much the printing of questionnaires will set the budget back. The difficulty tends to lie in the matter of whether the funding body (research funding bodies are discussed in the next section of this chapter) is willing to pay for equipment. A fair number of restrictions apply in this area: many funding bodies will not pay for computers, printers and the like; and equipment associated with clinical activities – for example an exercise treadmill, a piece of kit for an operating theatre, or a TENS machine – may be regarded as health service costs rather than research costs (see below for a further discussion of this tension between health service and research grant costs). Sometimes, when such costs will be met by the research grant giver, it will be necessary to stipulate into whose ownership the equipment will pass when the research is over. Usually there will be formal guidance from the grant-giving body on these matters, and there is generally someone there who will happily answer queries about their rules.

Services

Services, covering a wide range of activities, can be rather more difficult to estimate. Although establishing the fee for some essential training may be easy, the likely charges for a task like transcribing your interviews with patients may be tricky. How many interviews will there be? How long will they last? How do you want the transcripts set out? These decisions will need to be made if you are to get close to an accurate figure for the costs. But, if the interviews won't be complete and ready for transcribing until next year, who will be employed to do them? Often it will be a freelance person and you won't usually be able to fix a price with a specific person such a long time ahead. So it is with many of these costs. Good forward planning of the research activities – for timing and total numbers – together with best available current costs and some educated guessing will usually allow you to arrive at a reasonably accurate estimate which won't leave you short or with an embarrassing surplus at the finish. There are people in university departments and in health service R&D departments who will have available some indicative costs for common services such as transcribing.

Some charges for services can be impossible to gauge with any confidence. For example, we have more than once tried to guess how much money will be needed for a search by the UK's Office for National Statistics. In each case we were arranging to supply the Office with a list of patients who had been the subjects of an earlier clinical research project; the Office's job was to determine whether they had subsequently died and, if so, to supply us with the causes of the deaths. The snag is that the final costs depended on how many had died, and how easy it was to trace them (whether the computer can do it or whether a member of their staff needs to hand-search any databases). We can't accurately tell, when sending the lists, what these outcomes (and thereby charges) will be. You have to spend some time, calculating possible ranges of likely outcomes and set down for your prospective funders what you think the cost will be. And you cannot afford to underestimate because, once the work is done, these fees must be paid. You won't look very smart if your head of department gets an invoice which your budget, on close scrutiny, cannot meet. Fortunately, most costs for services are reasonably predictable – with sufficient care and attention to detail.

Salaries

You may plan to carry out your project either on your own or with a colleague or two, in your spare time or when you are allowed at your work to research rather than undertake patient care. If so, you may skip this section of the chapter – although you should read to the bottom of this paragraph before moving ahead. We are discussing here the application to funding bodies for the biggest costs of research – salaries of the staff who will do the work. Research is no different to other endeavours – staff salaries usually account for by far the largest expenditure. It is worth mentioning that when clinicians, other health service staff, or university employees are researching without any salary support then their employer is carrying substantial cost. A proportion of that person's salary and of all the other expenses associated with employing someone (pension, national insurance, space occupied, heating and lighting, indemnity insurance, and so on) is, in effect, being given free of charge by the employer to the research project.

Fortunately health organisations and higher education institutions are frequently willing to meet those concealed costs because the person undertaking the work is deemed to be developing professionally by doing the research. Over the last 20 years or so this relaxed environment has, however, been moving ever closer towards a system in which the true cost to an organisation of carrying out research must be determined, sought, and awarded up-front before the research is allowed to start. Most research in today's healthcare in the UK is funded through designated money that has been awarded after application to an external funding body.

When working out the costs for research staff you are likely to need some help; it is far from easy to do unassisted. Thankfully, most experienced researchers have been through the same process, perhaps many times. If you can approach or collaborate with one of these colleagues he or she may tell you that they, in turn, depend on the knowledge and skills of research administration staff in health services R&D departments or in university institutes. These are the people who can talk you through your plans for the project. What kind of researcher do you need, and from what (if any) clinical discipline? You might have unrealistic expectations about either the volume of work that someone can do or their ability to work with limited supervision; the colleagues who work in research administration can often spot when you are being over-optimistic about keeping salary costs down – they've seen it all before.

When applying for research grants we all want to keep these large staff costs down to a minimum: not because we don't want a large research grant but because we fear that a bottom-line figure for the project, if too great, will get the application rejected. Such misgivings are well founded but, on the other hand, the experienced researchers and administrators who deliberate on our applications can spot when the amount of work expected of some poor, as yet unidentified, research assistant is excessive and likely to prove impossible to accomplish.

Consultation, followed by careful time budgeting of the tasks will show you how long the whole project will last. A research assistant may not be needed for all stages of the work – employing someone once the project is underway or ending the employment once certain fieldwork tasks have been completed are ways of keeping costs down. To do this planning sensibly, you must be realistic about your own contribution. In particular, who will do the analysis and writing up of the findings? Prospective funders are all too familiar with projects where the fieldwork gets completed but the analysis or writing up is hopelessly delayed – even abandoned as the original researcher moves on to pastures new. Give careful thought to the time needed for analysis and writing up; if it will need more research staff time, you should include it in the application.

Although this book is about modest research projects, suitable for people early in their research careers, it is worth mentioning here that, in the funding of clinical trials, research grant awarding organisations do not usually expect to pay any of the costs associated with therapies. They regard these costs as ones that they can legitimately expect the health service to provide. For example, in a trial of family therapy versus routine treatment for young people who have self-harmed, the research organisation won't pay either for the treatment as usual or the family therapy – but it will fund: the creation of manuals that set out the exact form of therapies to be followed in the research, the cost of approaching potential participants, the random allocation, the research interviews before and after treatment, the careful scrutiny of the therapists' activity (to see that they have adhered to the manuals), the searching of health records to determine outcomes, the analysis of the data, and the publication and dissemination of the findings. The health service in the UK and elsewhere has a variety of procedures and organisations that can assist with the extra costs that the research adds to the clinical care of patients. These complex arrangements – which can apply in a similar way to studies involving diagnostic testing and illness screening – will not usually affect the early career researcher who is working at a rather smaller scale.

Transport

Setting out the cost for your travel and that of your co-researchers is straightforward. As with other calculations, it requires some attention to detail and then a final figure with some simple indications of how the costs are worked out. Don't forget that patients should sometimes be reimbursed for travel to research interviews or for any extra hospital visits resulting from their participation in the research.

Another area where travel costs can be incurred, perhaps more often in the larger projects, is in the reimbursement of the costs of service users and carers when they have agreed to be part of a research project's planning and monitoring committees (see Chapter 16). It is normal practice, and only fair, to ensure that they are not out of pocket. Lots of researchers don't think it reasonable to expect service users to give their time free – they are being used in a consultancy capacity and a modest fee for attending monitoring meetings is quite proper.

Publishing

A recent and growing form of publication of research findings is to pay for publication in an open access on-line journal. In one common form of this type of publishing, the authors pay a substantial fee (which can be many hundreds of US dollars) when submitting the research paper. The journal sets in train the peer review process and, once (or if) successfully revised, the paper is published in the on-line journal. At first sight this seems rather odd, especially if you are used to the idea that no money changes hands when you send your work to a conventional journal. Why would people pay to publish their work? Perhaps it might even seem a bit dodgy: would a journal turn down as many poor papers if authors were paying? Those authors (and their chums) might not be so likely to pay again next time. Might weaker papers be accepted through this process? The problem with conventional journals, however, is this: most of them are available only to people who pay a subscription to the professional body or publishing company who produce the journal. That means that the wider public, especially those who don't work in or close to a university (which is likely to subscribe to many of these journals), cannot readily and promptly get access to the published findings of the research. The large governmental research funding bodies have been increasingly unhappy about funding research which can only be viewed by people who have directly or indirectly paid for access to third party, largely commercial organisations. Open access journals mean that the taxpayers can see the research they paid for and so can people in lower income countries who might not be able to afford the subscriptions to conventional journals. Whatever the merits or shortcomings of fee-based, open access publication, publication fees are a legitimate addition to grant applications; some funding bodies have begun to insist on open access publication.

WHERE TO APPLY

There is a vast array of available grants for research so it can be daunting to embark on finding a suitable source of funds and then complete their application process. Two basic tips apply: look out for research calls specific to your area of work; and become familiar with one or more funding directories that draw together some of the many sources of funds.

Calls from charities and public bodies

Keep an eye out for calls for research in your area of interest. If a research funder puts out an advertisement stating that they are eager to fund research into the very topic that you want to pursue then this is too good a chance to miss. These calls can be quite specific or more general. This example (see Figure 15.1) is for a potentially substantial amount of money to support any of a designated range of research projects concerned with eye disease. Some calls might be more specific (only concerned, say, with interventions for acute glaucoma) while others might widen the topics set out here – to include any form of health care for eye disease.

Ophthalmic Research Funding Project Grants 2010

Guide Dogs is pleased to announce a call for ophthalmic research grant proposals. We are particularly interested in receiving high-quality scientific research proposals relating to the preservation and improvement of sight in people who are already visually impaired, and the epidemiology of ocular disease.

Proposals from heads of established ophthalmic units or research departments will be considered. Funds are available to cover staff, equipment and consumables for projects lasting up to three years. The level of support available will depend on the scientific needs of the work, but awards will not normally exceed £80k per annum.

Applicants are requested to submit an initial five-page application in line with Guide Dogs' application guidelines. Successful projects from this stage will be asked to provide a full proposal.

The closing date for initial applications is **Friday 19 February 2010**.

For further information you can download the 'Initial application form and guidelines'

[email address and telephone number for person to speak to supplied on original advertisement]

Guide Dogs

FIGURE 15.1   A call, through a journal advertisement, for applications to a charity for research funding.

The advertisement of a research funding award by the charity Guide Dogs is fairly typical of awards where substantial amounts of research funding are offered: it is in two stages. The first (outline) stage is not a very long document – although it can take some considerable time to prepare such an application. If you successfully negotiate the first stage in a process such as this one (perhaps waiting for two to three months for an answer), you will then be given something like a couple of months in which to prepare a longer and highly detailed description of the project. You might usually expect the funding body to seek substantially more peer review for the full proposal than for the outline.

At both stages the question being asked in the research will need to be set out clearly, together with the design, methods, measures, outcomes and plans for disseminating your findings. You will usually need to set out an estimated timeframe for all stages of the work. Alongside the technical description of the proposed research, many of these application forms have a separate section where the study must be described in terms suited to the non-expert, or lay person. This section will be one of the most important and care needs to be taken to describe very clearly what you plan in jargon-free terms, without patronising the reader. For help in writing this section we recommend the wealth of good advice offered by the Plain English Campaign; their free guide to writing plainly about medical information is a good starting point but there are many useful writing tips on their web site: http://www.plainenglish.co.uk/files/medicalguide.pdf

Even at the outline stage you will probably have to estimate your costs, perhaps breaking them down into categories such as salaries, expenses, equipment, and so on; at the full proposal stage these costs will be set out in detail.

On-line directories of research funding

We recommend becoming familiar with one or more of the on-line directories of research funding. In England one of the most useful is RDFunding, the National Health Service's own searchable website: www.rdfunding.org.uk/. The site forms part of the activities of the National Institute for Health Research. Although the site is oriented towards research in England it contains information and links for many funding organisations that will support research in other countries, especially the other three UK nations. The site is searchable and provides concise but incomplete information about potential funding – usually offering a link to the correct place on the funding body's own web site. As with all searching (see Chapter 2), a variety of terms may be needed to locate the best search results: Dinesh tried 'self-harm' in RDFunding but only found one database entry; when he tried 'suicide' instead, he found several potentially suitable sources of research awards for which his project might be suited.

Dinesh

In the event, Dinesh decided that all of the specific grants that he located were more suited to projects larger than the one that he was ready to get underway. His supervisor suggested that he look into the possibility of support from his own teaching hospital trust's charitable foundation. Many of the large teaching centres have such organisations – funded through local benefactors and vigorous fundraising. Such charitable foundations will usually expect to fund local research projects, normally ones that are not too large or costly. They are likely to be interested where there is a prospect that the research would lead, once completed, to the submission of a good proposal to one of the governmental or charitable funders for a large-scale study.

He has applied for funds to cover the costs of printing and copying his various measures, staff time to pay a clerical officer to collect and store completed forms in a safe place, access to the software he needs to store and handle his data, and a consultancy fee for the statistician who will help him analyse the results.

Anna

Anna is aware, from her emerging plan for her qualitative study, that she will incur some costs in carrying out and analysing her one-to-one interviews. She expects to record possibly 20 or so interviews – for which she will need a digital recorder with microphone. She will want to pay someone to transcribe the interviews on to paper, and she thinks she may want to purchase computer software (probably NVivo) for the analysis. She has spoken to the two medical executive directors – in public health and in primary care – in the NHS Primary Care Trust responsible for commissioning health care in her area. One of them has asked her to write to him with detailed estimates of her proposed costs (she has still to do the details but thinks she may need around £1000). He has indicated that he will probably be able to find the sum concerned because he is very keen to see progress in immunisation rates. Anna's research may help with improved procedures and policies; at the very least it should demonstrate that the Trust is actively seeking ways to achieve such improvements.

16

Getting Permission to Go Ahead

If you are to undertake research in the healthcare setting you will need permission and approval from several sources. The environment that demands such permission is constantly changing. In the UK, as recently as 2000, it was a more relaxed business than today although, following changes now in place, the process is probably more straightforward now than it was in the mid-2000s. Depending on what you plan to do in your research, you may very well need an ethical review of your plans. You may also need approval from healthcare trusts or hospitals. Honorary contracts may be needed for researchers who are not employed directly by the service where the data are collected; if your data are to come from more than one source, you may need an honorary contract with another healthcare organisation, or someone working with you on the project may need a contract to be arranged with your hospital or clinic.

These arrangements take time in at least two ways. The forms that must be filled out can take a good deal of time, and the deliberations made by others once you have submitted the application can take a while to come through (and may lead to demands for alterations or clarification of your proposal and further delay).

WILL MY RESEARCH NEED ETHICAL REVIEW?

This is a key question that will greatly affect the permission and formal application required before you can get started. There are many projects that you and others may think of as clinical research that might, nonetheless, be regarded by people of influence as either clinical audit or service evaluation, neither of which need go through the full procedure for ethics review. We have included here a useful guide produced for the UK's NHS National Research Ethics Service; it attempts the difficult task of separating out these three kinds of enquiry (see Figure 16.1). It can be used by prospective researchers at the design stage to help to determine whether a submission for ethical review will be required.

If the project fits the research category, there are some guidelines that can help with deciding what permissions are needed. Broadly speaking, ethical review by a Research Ethics Committee will be required in the UK if the potential participants in research are going to be identified because of their past or present use of UK health services or social care – whether they be patients, service users, or relatives or carers. It will usually be necessary to seek ethical review if the research involves collecting information or tissue from a user of health or social care services. In addition, when the research involves use of information or tissue that was previously obtained for earlier research or clinical reasons, ethical review will be required if there is any possibility of individuals being identified.

In the event, many research studies in the UK will need ethical review, which will usually be carried out by a local Research Ethics Committee (REC). The first step is to complete the on-line form – currently

---

Getting Started in Health Research, First Edition. David Bowers, Allan House and David Owens.
© 2011 David Bowers, Allan House and David Owens. Published 2011 by Blackwell Publishing Ltd.

DIFFERENTIATING AUDIT, SERVICE EVALUATION AND RESEARCH

RESEARCH	CLINICAL AUDIT	SERVICE EVALUATION
The attempt to derive generalisable new knowledge, including studies that aim to generate hypotheses, as well as studies that aim to test them.	Designed and conducted to produce information to inform delivery of best care.	Designed and conducted solely to define or judge current care.
Quantitative research – designed to test a hypothesis. Qualitative research – identifies/explores themes following established methodology.	Designed to answer the question: "Does this service reach a predetermined standard?"	Designed to answer the question: "What standard does this service achieve?"
Addresses clearly defined questions, aims and objectives.	Measures against a standard.	Measures current service without reference to a standard.
Quantitative research – may involve evaluating or comparing interventions, particularly new ones. Qualitative research – usually involves studying how interventions and relationships are experienced.	Involves an intervention in use ONLY (the choice of treatment is that of the clinician and patient according to guidance, professional standards and/or patient preference.)	Involves an intervention in use ONLY (the choice of treatment is that of the clinician and patient according to guidance, professional standards and/or patient preference.)
Usually involves collecting data that are additional to those for routine care but may include data collected routinely. May involve treatments, samples or investigations additional to routine care.	Usually involves analysis of existing data but may include administration of simple interview or questionnaire.	Usually involves analysis of existing data but may include administration of simple interview or questionnaire.
Quantitative research - study design may involve allocating patients to intervention groups. Qualitative research uses a clearly defined sampling framework underpinned by conceptual or theoretical justifications.	No allocation to intervention groups: the healthcare professional and patient have chosen intervention before clinical audit.	No allocation to intervention groups: the healthcare professional and patient have chosen intervention before service evaluation.
May involve randomisation	No randomisation	No randomisation
ALTHOUGH ANY OF THESE THREE MAY RAISE ETHICAL ISSUES, UNDER CURRENT GUIDANCE:-		
RESEARCH REQUIRES REC REVIEW	AUDIT DOES NOT REQUIRE REC REVIEW	SERVICE EVALUATION DOES NOT REQUIRE REC REVIEW

FIGURE 16.1   A helpful guide to distinguishing between research, clinical audit and service evaluation.

available on the web site of the National Research Ethics Service (NRES) at www.nres.npsa.nhs.uk. This can be a lengthy and detailed procedure but at least the single form (the Integrated Research Application System, IRAS form) is used for a variety of the permissions needed; all being well you should not need to fill in separate forms for various other bodies who may wish to check out and approve your plans. In the UK the other official body likely to require your application for scrutiny and approval is the Research and Development (R&D) department of your local hospital or primary care trust; they will use this integrated form. In larger and more complex studies there may be requirements to seek permission from governmental bodies that deal with such diverse matters as research where there is use of radioactive substances, gene therapy, or data collected with neither consent nor anonymisation; these steps are not ones usually taken by someone who is starting out on research, and won't be discussed here any further (but can be accessed through the NRES web site, above).

For the ethical review form you will need to summarise the study in a number of ways. For example, you will have to describe the study briefly so that a member of the public will understand it. Dinesh's account, written in less than 300 words is shown in Figure 16.2.

Please provide a brief summary of the research (maximum 300 words) using language easily understood by lay reviewers and members of the public. This summary will be published on the website of the National Research Ethics Service following the ethical review.

Each year around 150,000 people attend emergency departments in England because of self-harm, many of them attending more than once. On 80% of occasions the person has self-poisoned, usually by taking an overdose of a medicine; around 20% of the time the patient has self-injured, usually by intentionally cutting himself or herself.

People who attend hospital because of self-harm receive a variable standard of care. This is a weakness in the NHS that the NICE guideline on self-harm openly admits to. Many patients are not assessed for their psychological needs, and little psychological therapy is offered. Many people leave the emergency department before their assessment and treatment is complete. Reports from staff and patients suggest high rates of dissatisfaction with the service provided.

Despite many patients repeating self-harm over the weeks and months that follow, there is no clear evidence about what could be done to reduce this repetition. Improving the experience of the care received might lead to better outcomes. One plausible improvement is delivery of an advocacy service – providing patients who wish it with the help of another person who will act personally for them while in the emergency department: helping, for example, in giving and receiving information and in making decisions.

The study will describe rates of attendance, early departure, and six-month reattendance for adults attending one emergency department after self-harm. Patients who are sufficiently conscious and alert, and who consent to take part, will be asked about their mood, their satisfaction with services, and their interest in an advocacy service – if one were available. Firm evidence about any benefits of an advocacy service will need to come out of a randomised controlled trial. The present study will provide information that will be essential if such a trial is to be set up.

FIGURE 16.2   Dinesh's summary of his research for a lay audience.

It is quite usual for this brief summary to be placed, once approval has been given, on the web site of the ethics service – there for all to see, probably for several years.

Of course, elsewhere on the form, you will need to describe parts of the proposed study at greater length. You must set out the main ethical and design issues – and explain how you have addressed them. Below is an extract from Anna's draft application for ethical approval – from the section describing these matters (see Figure 16.3).

Please summarise the main ethical and design issues arising from the study and say how you have addressed them.

The study is a cross-sectional observational study. It seeks to find out about experience, knowledge and opinion concerning MMR (measles, mumps and rubella) vaccine from mothers of children eligible for the first dose of the vaccine – at around 13 months of the child's age. The study aims to improve our understanding of the factors that influence uptake of the vaccination for children. It will do so by inviting mothers to take part in a one-to-one semi-structured interview, and the data collected will be analysed qualitatively. The plan for the study has been drawn up following consultation with members of the existing patient group that meets regularly in the general practice where the research will take place.

I, the applicant for this IRAS process, will undertake all of the interviewing and I will identify the study population of eligible mothers from the lists of patients at the practice where I work as a General Practitioner. I plan to sample the study population in a purposive way, using quotas (see below). I will approach mothers directly when they are at the surgery for routine childcare visits. I will explain verbally the purpose of the project and the invitation to take part. I will, on the same occasion, give the mother a written explanation of the project and her proposed involvement (see Subject Information Leaflet). I will arrange to speak with her over the following week on the telephone to establish whether she is willing to take part. The written material already given to the mother will incorporate the consent form (see Informed Consent Form). I will make an appointment with a consenting mother to meet me for the interview, and she and I will complete the consent form together before beginning the interview. [**Note: we haven't established when in the child's vaccination cycle the approach would be made: should go into protocol and here. Discuss in team**]

The interviews will be in the form of a semi-structured interview, estimated as lasting for 40–50 minutes. I will offer interview at the surgery or at the participant's home, according to her preference. The next paragraph summarises the nature of the questions in the semi-structured interview. I will explain, from the first conversation when approaching the mother, that the interviews will be audio-recorded and transcribed. I will, as soon as I have obtained written consent to take part, explain the audio-recording and the separate written consent to the recording and transcribing (see Informed Consent Form: Audio-recording Annex), and the arrangements for storage and destruction of the recording and transcript …

Continued …

FIGURE 16.3   Anna's provisional summary of the ethical challenges in her research.

You will be asked to state the nature of your principal research question or objective and of any secondary ones; once again these statements should be set out in language comprehensible to a member of the public.

You will have realised by this point that there is substantial repetition in the filling out of these kinds of applications for permission (and for funding). Points that you have already made must be repeated, perhaps in more detail, or in more lay terms. Some of this rather repetitive procedure is, however, undoubtedly useful for you. You will find, again and again, once the study is underway that you have to tell colleagues and friends (and other people interested in how you are spending your time, such as your seniors) what you are trying to achieve with the project. Getting the main question and the scientific explanation of your work into a short, snappy and accurate but jargon-free outline is essential. Only in this way will you seem to be spending your efforts (and those of study participants) effectively.

What is the principal research question/objective? *Please put this in language comprehensible to a lay person.*

Is it feasible to plan a randomised controlled trial that determines whether an advocacy service for people attending the emergency department because of self-harm would prove effective, judged by a reduction in repetition of self-harm?

What are the secondary research questions/objectives if applicable? *Please put this in language comprehensible to a lay person.*

The study will determine numbers of patients attending one emergency department in a teaching hospital because of self-harm, and the rate of repetition at six months. Also determined will be the proportion of such patients who remain sufficiently long (do not leave before assessment and treatment are reasonably complete) and are sufficiently alert to be potentially assisted by an advocacy service while in the emergency department. Patients' mood and satisfaction with services will also be measured.

In a sample of these patients, the study will investigate opinions about the current service for people who have self-harmed, and the acceptability of an advocacy service, if one were available.

FIGURE 16.4   Dinesh's research question as presented on a research ethics form.

Ethical review forms generally ask for considerable detail about how participants, especially if they are patients, will be recruited and dealt with once in the study. The form will ask you for details about how people will be identified – particularly asking whether you will be using routinely collected information, and who will be doing the identification (is it a researcher or someone already in the clinical team?). This is because there are greater concerns now than there used to be about access to such sources of clinical data. Generally speaking, permission to identify people is obtained more easily if the procedure is carried out mainly or wholly by the healthcare team already dealing with the care of those patients.

The ethical review committee will want to know whether you plan to obtain consent for participation and, if so, precisely how you plan to do so. You will need to submit, with your ethical review form, copies of your proposed participants' information sheet and consent form; Anna's first draft versions are included as annexes to this chapter. Anna plans to make audio-recordings, so she will need also to write a separate form (not annexed here) for permission to do so, stating what will happen to the recording and its transcription – in terms of storage and making the recording and the transcript as anonymous as possible. We have more to say about anonymisation and confidentiality of data in Chapter 18.

In the case of research where no consent is to be sought, you will have to take particular care to explain why not; the default position is that consent is generally required. If you are using routinely obtained, existing health-service information about patients, ethical approval is more likely to be obtained readily if the data are to be anonymised at the point of your collection.

You must be ready to make clear, in the application form, in the protocol, and on patient information leaflets, exactly what will happen to research participants in your study – including how many times things will be done to them: when you will try to recruit them, how you will gain consent (often allowing time for people to reconsider), what will be the timing of any interviews, and when any tests, treatments or interventions will take place. Many studies incorporate follow-up of some kind and this procedure will need to be explained and its timing included.

As we have suggested throughout this book, it is good practice to involve users of services, patients, carers, members of the public and the like in the planning of research. This stage, the setting out of the detailed plans for the study's participants, is especially an area for such involvement, and the form will ask you about whether you have done so.

RESEARCH GOVERNANCE

It is essential that all the necessary paperwork for the project is kept in order. All necessary permissions must not only be obtained but must be documented and kept up to date. Part of the approval process undertaken in the IRAS form (above) will result in registration of the research with an R&D department – in a hospital trust, or primary care trust, or other health-service organisation. This department may well wish to audit their own and your procedures. At any time, at short notice, they may require you to demonstrate that all of your permissions and processes are as they should be. Consequently, honorary contracts, ethical reports, reports to funding bodies, and any other requirements must have actually been carried out – and you must hold the documents that confirm that it is so. Our top tip is to keep all of these items together in a file, with a front sheet that will remind you of renewal dates or due dates for despatching any reports that are stipulated requirements of your research (see examples in appendix).

APPENDIX

Greendale Health Centre official headed paper, with logo and address

MMR Uptake Study

A research project investigating mothers' opinions about agreeing to MMR vaccination for their child

MOTHER'S INFORMATION SHEET AND CONSENT FORM

A large-print version of this sheet is available on request

You have been invited to take part in a research project called the MMR Uptake Study. Before you decide whether to accept, we would like to explain why the research is being done and what it will involve. Please read this information carefully, and discuss it with others if you wish. Ask us if anything is unclear, or if you would like more information.

Take time to decide whether or not you wish to take part.

Thank you for reading this information sheet.

What is the purpose of the study?

Although the health service recommends that children aged around one year receive MMR vaccine not all parents agree that their child should be vaccinated with MMR. In this research we are trying to find out what influences parents' decisions – to go ahead or to decline the vaccine for their child.

What is MMR vaccination?

The vaccine is a combined vaccine (three vaccines given together) that aims at protecting children against measles, mumps and rubella (German measles). It is usually given by injection to children around the age of 13 months, with a second dose given between the ages of three and five years to cover any children who haven't responded to the first dose.

Why have I been chosen?

You have been chosen because this research project is asking mothers in our general practice about their views on the vaccination and the way that we arrange for it to be given to the children in the practice. We will be asking other mothers to take part too – with a plan to include around 16 mothers in total.

Do we have to take part?

No, the MMR uptake study is entirely voluntary and you must to be happy to get involved before you agree to take part. If you decide that you might want to take part, you will be given this information sheet to keep. You will be asked later to sign consent forms but, even after that point, you will still be free to withdraw at any time and without giving a reason. If you decide not to take part, your doctor or the practice nurse will be happy to talk through any questions that you may have about the vaccination. Your son's or daughter's treatment and care will not be affected in any way.

What will happen to me if I take part?

If you are interested in taking part Dr Anna Flaxis will telephone you during the next week to see if you have made your mind up to take part. If you have, we will make an appointment either for you to come to the surgery or for Dr Flaxis to come and visit you at home. She will be able to answer any questions you have and then if you are still interested you will be asked to sign the consent form (which you can see at the end of this document) to confirm that you are willing to take part.

After you have signed your consent form, Dr Flaxis will ask you some questions and record the conversation, which she will later have typed out. She will use the transcripts from the interviews of everyone in the study to summarise the opinions of mothers about the vaccination. We expect your interview to last about 45 minutes.

What will happen if my son or daughter has not had the MMR vaccine?

We are asking mothers to take part in the study after they have made their decision about the vaccination of their child. Our sample of mothers may therefore include some whose children have been vaccinated and some whose children have not.

What will I have to do after a research interview with the doctor?

This research only involves one interview. There won't be any request for a later, follow-up contact about the research.

What if my son or daughter needs other treatment while I am taking part in the research?

Being part of the research won't stop your son or daughter having any other treatment that your nurse or GP thinks he or she needs.

What are the possible disadvantages and risks of taking part?

We do not expect there will be any additional risk in taking part.

What are the possible benefits of taking part?

If you take part it will be after you have made your decision about MMR vaccination for your child. The research will not, therefore, have any direct benefit to you or your child. The main benefit is that the research project will help us learn more about how to help other people in the future with their decisions about vaccination.

What if there is a problem or something goes wrong?

If anything about your son's or daughter's treatment or health worries you, you can talk about it with the practice nurse or your general practitioner (family doctor).

If you have a concern about any aspect of this study, you should ask to speak with the researcher who will do her best to answer your questions (Telephone Number: . . .). If you remain unhappy you may wish to contact your local Patient Advice and Liaison Service (PALS, Telephone Number: . . .) or if you wish to complain formally you can do this through the NHS Complaints Procedure. Details can be obtained from the practice or any hospital.

There are no special compensation arrangements in place for this study. You may have grounds for legal action for compensation as a result of someone's negligence but you may have to pay for it. The normal NHS complaints mechanisms will still be available to you (if appropriate).

Will our taking part be kept confidential?

If you decide to participate in this research project, the information collected about you and your son or daughter during the course of the study will be kept strictly confidential. This information will be securely stored at the general practice on paper and electronically, under the provisions of the 1998 Data Protection Act. The researcher at the practice (one of the doctors there, Dr Flaxis) will hold a copy of the consent forms that you sign, which will have your name, address, phone number(s) and email address (if you have one) so that they can contact you about the study when needed. This information will not be accessed by any other personnel. Every effort will be made to ensure that any further information about you and your son or daughter will have your names and address removed so that you cannot be recognised from it. You will be allocated a study number, which will be used as a code to identify you on all study forms. Only the researcher herself will be able to identify you from this number.

Involvement of your General Practitioner (GP) / Family Doctor

With your permission your GP and the other clinicians at the practice involved in your son / daughter's care, will be kept informed, but otherwise all information about his / her treatment will remain confidential.

Who is organising and funding the research?

The Medical Director of the local Primary Care Trust (Greendale Health) has partly funded this project as it is seen as an important area for research. The rest of the cost of running it is being met by Greendale Health Centre who will be responsible for the organisation and running of the project.

Who has reviewed the study?

All research is looked at by an independent group of people called a Research Ethics Committee, to protect the safety, rights, well-being and dignity of those taking part. This study has been reviewed and approved by Greendale Research Ethics Committee.

What will happen if I do not want to carry on with the study?

If you withdraw consent from participation in the study after agreeing to take part, any information collected from you for the study will be withdrawn from the final study analysis.

What will happen to the results of the study?

When the study is complete the results will be published in a medical journal, but no individual participants will be identified. If you would like to obtain a copy of the published results, please ask Dr Flaxis or any of the nurses or doctors in the practice.

Contact Details

If you have any questions or would like more information you can speak to the researcher or to your doctor or the practice nurse. Contact details are:

[insert contact details for relevant local contacts]

Mother's Consent Form for the MMR Uptake Study

A research project investigating mothers' opinions about agreeing to MMR vaccination for their child

Participant ID:	Initials:
Child's date of birth:	Principal Investigator:

Please initial after each question

1. I confirm that I have read and understand the information sheet for the above study and have had the opportunity to ask questions.   . . . .

2. I understand that participation is voluntary and that I am free to withdraw at any time without my care or that of my child or any legal rights being affected.   . . . .

3. I understand that my child's medical record may be looked at by the researcher to collect data for the purposes of this study.   . . . .

4. I understand that if I withdraw from the above study, the data collected from me will not be used in analysing the results of the study. I understand that my identity will remain anonymous.   . . . .

5. I agree to allow any information or results arising from this study to be used for healthcare and/or medical research purposes. I understand that my identity will remain anonymous.   . . . .

6. I agree that my son / daughter's GP and other clinicians treating him / her at the practice, will be notified of our participation in this study.   . . . .

7. I agree to take part in the study   . . . .

_____   _____   _____

Name of participant   Date   Signature

_____   _____   _____

Name of Person taking consent   Date   Signature

(1 copy for participant; 1 for the CTRU; original stored in Investigator Site File)

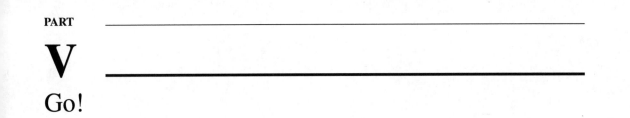

Go!

17

Recruiting the Participants

In Chapter 16 we considered the permissions needed to go ahead with a research project. These official procedures are, however, not the end of the story as far as the practicalities are concerned. In the event, how are you going to approach and recruit the participants in your study? It might happen entirely in your own clinic or surgery or treatment room, in which case it will be down to your own charm and powers of persuasion. More often, the first practical step in recruitment of participants will be the gaining of cooperation from others in the health service.

WORKING WITH THE HEALTHCARE SYSTEM

There are a number of ways in which people participate in health research. Some are approached directly for their agreement and consent to take part, while others participate without making contact face to face – when it is clinical material such as that found in their case notes, radiographs or lung-function tests that form the sample for study. Although the matter of permission can differ considerably depending on whether individual consent is sought (see Chapter 16), in discussing studies where data are collected without individual consent, we will assume here that the permission has been properly obtained.

Recruitment of your sample of participants will depend on your detailed knowledge of the healthcare system as it functions in your part of the organisation. If, for example, you want to recruit patients who have attended the emergency department (ED) because of ankle injury, it might very well be the emergency department's administrative staff who will determine your path to success. You might want each patient who attends because of ankle injury to be identified and asked particular questions during their consultation. If so, you might be able to arrange for the ED clerical staff who are booking the patients into the department to identify these people and attach your short questionnaire to the blank ED record – so that the doctor or nurse seeing the patient will ask and record the answers to those questions while undertaking the consultation. Alternatively, you might want to carry out a qualitative study of the experience of acute ankle injury, hospital care, treatment, follow-up and outcome. To do so you will need to approach the patients for their consent to meet with you. ED reception staff might be willing to attach an initial consent sheet to the case record when the patients book in to the ED; if they do, the nurse or doctor dealing with the patient's case could ask simply whether the person was willing to be telephoned by you to discuss taking part. Another approach entirely might be a plan to collect all the records of people who recently attended because of ankle injury and to make an epidemiological analysis of their characteristics and care pathways, perhaps comparing people who did and didn't have their ankle X-rayed.

Getting Started in Health Research, First Edition. David Bowers, Allan House and David Owens.
© 2011 David Bowers, Allan House and David Owens. Published 2011 by Blackwell Publishing Ltd.

In all of these notional examples it is plain that the recruitment of participants will depend largely on your ability to recruit the help of the administrative staff in the ED. You will need to gain the support for your work from the relevant manager of the administrative staff, and the staff who work at ED reception themselves, if they are to be consistent in carrying out the tasks that will enable your research. Clinicians too will need gentle persuasion if they are to make the small extra efforts that you require. Successful recruitment in research is not just the face-to-face work with individual patients or clients; success rests on intimate knowledge of the system and the roles of key personnel, and on your effective negotiations with the people who are going to help you to recruit, or going to collect data on your behalf.

Earlier in the book we drew attention to the increasing collaboration between researchers and service users and carers. Service users are well placed to help you prepare your procedures regarding recruitment of potential participants, pointing out what is likely to be an attractive or aversive line of approach: When is a good or bad time to talk with patients or hand them leaflets? Will it depend on their particular condition or predicament? How quickly or slowly might you follow up an initial approach – to clinch the deal on participation? Would people prefer to see you in clinic while already there at a routine visit or visit you on a separate occasion? Should you offer home, clinic, or somewhere else as the venue for data collection?

DOCUMENTATION

There are many good reasons for paying close attention to the written material that will be used in the recruitment process. It may be very useful to have attractively laid out leaflets or fact sheets that explain the purpose of your research. In many projects, there will need to be patient information leaflets for the consent stage (see Chapter 16) but this is not the only place for paper resources about the research. Well-written and effectively presented information will help convince those colleagues who are willing to approach their patients and invite them to take part. This is another area of preparation that may be assisted greatly by incorporating service users and carers into the drafting and laying out of the documents.

A more contemporary approach to this kind of information and advertisement of research is the provision of web sites that offer potential participants further information, Frequently Asked Questions (FAQs), and the like. Such sites may, as well as addressing potential recruits, offer further information and support to people who have gone a stage further and are already recruited as participants to the research.

Creating a web site for the research is plainly not something that a researcher in a small study can undertake. But the larger research organisations are increasingly involved with this kind of advance in the provision of information. For example, Cancer Research UK display a great deal of information in their web site's Patient Information section concerning research – especially with regard to clinical trials, as this extract (from February 2011) shows (www.cancerhelp.org.uk/trials/taking-part/index.htm) (Figure 17.1).

Look at what the site offers in relation to someone's interest in taking part in a trial: advantages and disadvantages of taking part, privacy, the science associated with the way the results will be set out, and so on. On other pages they suggest questions that a patient who is thinking about or is actually taking part in a trial might ask the research team. The information in the trials database is written in plain English for patients, their families and friends. It includes details of trials supported by a wide range of organisations, not just Cancer Research UK.

This kind of information for participants, more usually on paper than on the web, has multiple purposes. It sets out the merits of the research and provides essential details, such as the names and addresses and contact details of the research team, explanations of any procedures, estimated duration of interviews, procedures for claiming reimbursement for travel, and progress with the study. A study web site might ultimately attach final reports on the findings and their implications.

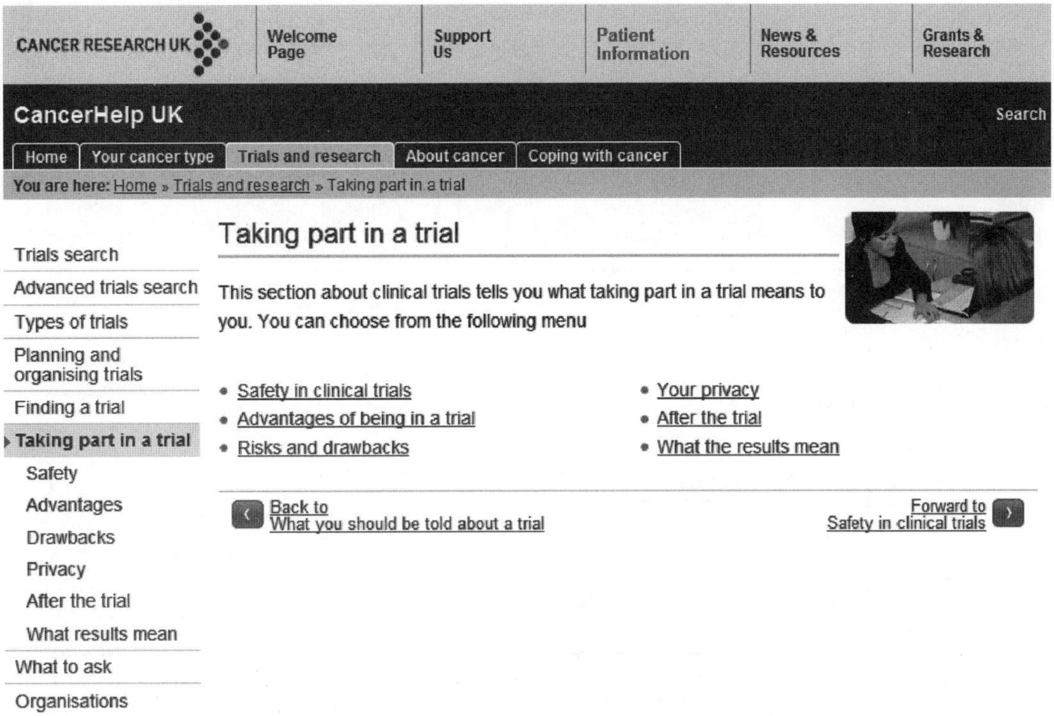

| CANCER RESEARCH UK | Welcome Page | Support Us | Patient Information | News & Resources | Grants & Research |

CancerHelp UK Search

| Home | Your cancer type | Trials and research | About cancer | Coping with cancer |

You are here: Home » Trials and research » Taking part in a trial

Trials search

Advanced trials search

Types of trials

Planning and organising trials

Finding a trial

▸ **Taking part in a trial**

  Safety

  Advantages

  Drawbacks

  Privacy

  After the trial

  What results mean

What to ask

Organisations

Taking part in a trial

This section about clinical trials tells you what taking part in a trial means to you. You can choose from the following menu

- Safety in clinical trials
- Advantages of being in a trial
- Risks and drawbacks

- Your privacy
- After the trial
- What the results mean

‹ Back to
What you should be told about a trial

Forward to ›
Safety in clinical trials

FIGURE 17.1   An example of a clinical research web site aimed at potential participants in one or more study.

WALKING THOUGH THE RECRUITMENT PROCEDURE

Putting aside research that focuses on case records or other routinely collected data, where study participants are to be invited – one by one – to take part it is a good idea to 'walk through' the steps that will be taken by the potential participants and by the research team.

Dinesh

Dinesh has a clear idea, from the experience of his day job as a nurse in the emergency department, about the usual pathways that patients follow when attending the emergency department because of self-harm. He draws a flow diagram – an 'algorithm' or sequence of steps resulting from decisions by the patient and staff (Figure 17.2). He knows to include not only the decisions made by staff but also those where patients decide to leave the emergency department before their assessment and treatment has been completed.

When he has finished thinking through and drawing the main pathways he makes further jottings on the diagram (Figure 17.2) where he thinks that advocacy might be useful in real clinical practice – if such a service were in place. For the planning of his basic descriptive study he can use this 'walk through' of the patients' differing journeys through care. It will help him to ensure that he collects data at the most important points, not ignoring potential losses at certain stages of some patients' care. He also has to decide at which point (or points) in the pathway he will ask a sample of patients whether they would consider advocacy. You will recall that he plans to enquire about the views of patients who would, in similar circumstances, be eligible were there to be a future clinical trial to judge the merits of advocacy.

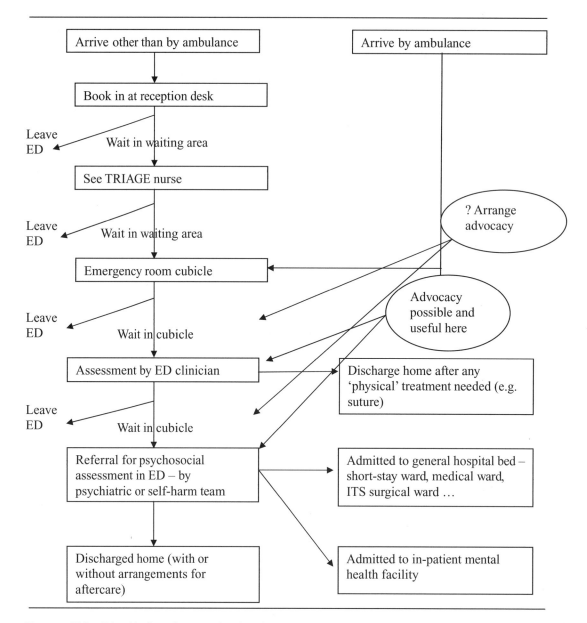

FIGURE 17.2 Dinesh's flow diagram of patients' potential flows through the emergency department, and where advocacy might be introduced (real numbers of patients still to be added).

NON-PARTICIPATION

In quantitative research, at least, we expect our research sample of participants to represent the population. Only if this notion is true can the study's findings, based as they are on the estimates drawn from the sample, be held as true of the wider population. Consequently, it is important to those who appraise the quality of the research (peer reviewers, editors, thesis examiners, readers of the final papers) that there is an adequate description of who did and didn't take part. Not taking part in research is thereby of great

Health and disease in 85 year olds: baseline findings from the Newcastle 85+ cohort study

Joanna Collerton, *principal clinical rese arch fellow*[1], **Karen Davies**, *research nurse ma nager*[1], **Carol Jagger**, *professor of epidemiology*[1,2], **Andrew Kingston**, *research assistant (medical statistics)*[1], **John Bond**, *professor of social gerontology and health services research*[1,3], **Martin P Eccles**, *William Leech professor of primary care research*[1,3], **Louise A Robinson**, *professor of primary care and ageing*[1,3], **Carmen Martin-Ruiz**, *senior research associate*[1], **Thomasvon Zglinicki**, *professor of cellular gerontology*[1], **Oliver F W Ja mes**, *senior research fellow*[1], **Thomas B L Kirkwood**, *director*[1]

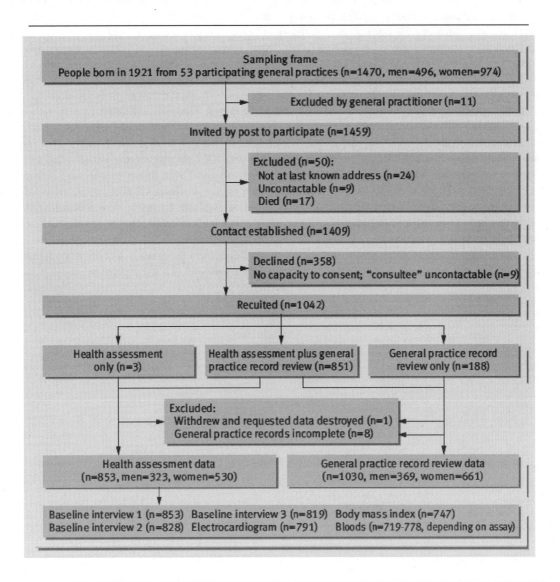

FIGURE 17.3   An example of a flow diagram from a published descriptive study.

interest. How many (what proportion) of the people eligible to take part actually did so? How many were approached but refused, or started but dropped out, and so on? Published studies sometimes (not often enough) set these matters out for the reader, often in the form of a flow chart (Figure 17.3). These diagrams are most commonly seen in clinical trials but can be just as useful in non-experimental studies, such as the one shown here.

It is worth commenting that, if your research project is going to make a good job of describing the relation between the study sample and the study population, it will be essential to collect the necessary data at all stages of the research. Part of the 'walk through' described above should include the putting in place of procedures to count and record the way in which potential participants do or do not become involved in the final research sample. Put another way, Dinesh will need to fill in the numbers for most of the steps in his algorithm (Figure 17.2) if he is to produce, for the final account of his completed study, a worthwhile diagram along the lines of the one shown in Figure 17.3.

In qualitative research little attention is generally given to the matter of non-participation, or refusal to take part. In a purposive sampling plan (Chapter 8) for example, target characteristics are set for the key criteria looked for in participants. People are then invited to take part in interviews, perhaps with a notional idea of carrying out up to a certain number of interviews – a number that might be in single figures for simple questions, rather more for more complicated enquiries. The plan will often be that, once the study is underway, the interviews will proceed until new categories of experience, themes or explanations stop arising; interviewing will then stop because data saturation has occurred (see Chapter 11). When someone turns down the offer to participate, this refusal is generally ignored and the next eligible person is approached instead. Any clearly apparent characteristics of people who refuse to take part are rarely described in the written accounts of such studies. It is good practice, however, to record some information about people contacted who were ineligible (and why), and any common themes evident concerning those who were eligible but declined to participate. This information helps to set the findings in the real-world context of the study population.

The next chapter will go on to deal with the collection of data from these study participants – the ones who have been identified and, where appropriate, been approached and given their consent.

18

Collecting and Recording the Data

Many clinical research projects are undertaken using routinely collected health data – such as case records, computerised monitoring registers, and the like. In research of this kind there is no need to deal with study participants face to face. In the first section of this chapter we will consider matters of collecting and recording these data. How to collect data directly from participants is dealt with later in the chapter.

DATA COLLECTION FORMS

Most researchers find it useful to set up a data collection form so that exactly the same data items are collected in every case. For example, Dinesh has started to set up the data collection sheet that he thinks he will need when he scrutinises the emergency department (ED) records of people who have attended after self-harm. Figure 18.1 shows the first page of his draft data collection sheet. On it he aims to collect, for each person attending ED because of self-harm, the basic data about socio-demographic factors and nature of the self-harm.

CODING OF VARIABLES

In a quantitative project such as the one that Dinesh is undertaking the data collected will be analysed using a computer. For this analysis, health researchers may well use computer software specifically designed for this purpose: SPSS, Stata, and Minitab are the three that we have found to be the best suited, and they are among the most widely used. For any of these computer applications, the data need to be coded in the kind of way shown in Figure 18.1. When using paper sheets like the one shown here, the researcher writes the data on to the forms, one by one while he or she is in the clinical area, then enters (types) these data into the computer later when back in the office.

Take as an example the matter of whether the patient who has come to the emergency department because of self-harm has attended as a result of self-poisoning (usually a medicine overdose), or self-injury (usually self-cutting), or both of these actions at the same time. The simplest way to record which one of these possibilities has occurred is to code the possibilities as three different (and arbitrary) numbers – say, 1 (self-poisoning), 2 (self-injury), and 3 (both, combined). A widely used procedure, as Dinesh has used here, is to provide a box into which he can write the correct code once he has scrutinised the clinical record to find out which method of self-harm was used by the patient. In these days of readily available computer expertise, paper coding sheets may sometimes be avoided and computer databases set up instead – to accept these codes in one step – but the principle is the same. Where the computer is

Getting Started in Health Research, First Edition. David Bowers, Allan House and David Owens.
© 2011 David Bowers, Allan House and David Owens. Published 2011 by Blackwell Publishing Ltd.

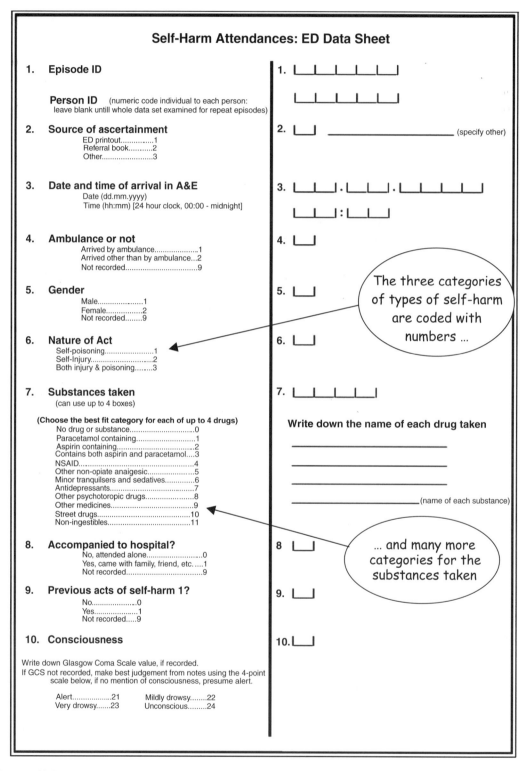

Self-Harm Attendances: ED Data Sheet

1. **Episode ID**

    Person ID   (numeric code individual to each person:
    leave blank untill whole data set examined for repeat episodes)

2. **Source of ascertainment**
    ED printout...............1
    Referral book...........2
    Other.......................3

3. **Date and time of arrival in A&E**
    Date (dd.mm.yyyy)
    Time (hh:mm) [24 hour clock, 00:00 - midnight]

4. **Ambulance or not**
    Arrived by ambulance....................1
    Arrived other than by ambulance...2
    Not recorded.................................9

5. **Gender**
    Male...................1
    Female.................2
    Not recorded........9

6. **Nature of Act**
    Self-poisoning.......................1
    Self-Injury............................2
    Both injury & poisoning........3

7. **Substances taken**
    (can use up to 4 boxes)

    (Choose the best fit category for each of up to 4 drugs)
    No drug or substance.............................0
    Paracetamol containing...........................1
    Aspirin containing...............................2
    Contains both aspirin and paracetamol....3
    NSAID...4
    Other non-opiate anaigesic....................5
    Minor tranquilsers and sedatives.............6
    Antidepressants.................................7
    Other psychotoropic drugs.....................8
    Other medicines.....................................9
    Street drugs..10
    Non-ingestibles....................................11

8. **Accompanied to hospital?**
    No, attended alone.........................0
    Yes, came with family, friend, etc......1
    Not recorded...................................9

9. **Previous acts of self-harm 1?**
    No....................0
    Yes...................1
    Not recorded.....9

10. **Consciousness**

    Write down Glasgow Coma Scale value, if recorded.
    If GCS not recorded, make best judgement from notes using the 4-point
    scale below, if no mention of consciousness, presume alert.

    Alert..................21   Mildly drowsy........22
    Very drowsy.......23   Unconscious.........24

1. |__|__|__|__|__|

   |__|__|__|__|__|

2. |__| _____ (specify other)

3. |__|__|__| . |__|__| . |__|__|__|__|

   |__|__| : |__|__|

4. |__|

5. |__|

6. |__|

The three categories of types of self-harm are coded with numbers ...

7. |__|__|__|__|

   Write down the name of each drug taken

   _____

   _____

   _____

   _____ (name of each substance)

... and many more categories for the substances taken

8 |__|

9. |__|

10. |__|

FIGURE 18.1   First page of Dinesh's draft coding sheet.

used there will usually be a restricted and specific choice to be made for the coding of each variable (or characteristic) included in the study.

Where Dinesh's close scrutiny of a clinical record doesn't reveal the method of self-harm, he can leave the box blank. Blank boxes, however, can lead to problems with the sequence of numbers that are later entered into the computer; there is a danger that the missing value might be ignored and the value for the next variable thereby mistaken for the missing one. Consequently, we usually give missing values a number of their own (another arbitrary number), often choosing a value not too close to the real options; here he chose the number 9 (a common choice for missing values). Missing values are considered in more detail below.

The above example, categorising the method of self-harm, had three possible values, each one mutually exclusive. Many variables offer only an alternative: yes or no, present or absent. Examples might be: male/female, previous episode or not, recently taken alcohol or not, and so on.

Less often, there are multiple possibilities (where more than one answer can be given). There are various ways of dealing with this difficulty (multiple categories are a good deal less straightforward in the analysis, so 'difficulty' is a fair word). We favour the reasonably simple method of setting out the categories, as before, but then offering more than one box to fill in. In this way, for example, Dinesh provided for the coding of each patient who self-poisoned: any patient could be easily coded for up to four separate categories of medicines (or, occasionally the taking of a non-ingestible substance). If the episode was not one of self-poisoning, all four boxes are coded zero. If only one medicine was taken, three of the boxes are coded zero. Dinesh uses zeros here because these values are not missing – there were simply no drugs taken. If the person (very unusually) took five medicines, he will ignore the drug that he deems to be the most trivial; this step introduces a small amount of data loss but causes no real problem provided that the rules for coding are established, and passed on to anyone else who becomes involved with the coding.

What we don't recommend is to categorise a metric or ordinal variable before coding it. Age is metric but could be recorded in bands (16–25, 26–35, etc.). Although Dinesh might feel sure that he will use such bands in the analysis, he should record the age and deal with the banding later – at the analysis stage. The software that we all use for data analysis readily chops variables into bands at our whim. You can change your mind and have different bands (fewer, more, different boundaries to the categories, and so on). The data are rendered imprecise by this kind of banding process (for instance, in banded coding of this kind ages 16 and 25 would be regarded as just the same when they differ a good deal); it may be that you won't need precise values when you come to analyse the data but you will throw away the possibility of altering your choice of categories if you categorise too early. In fact, in this case, Dinesh simply records date of birth; with that information, the software can easily calculate ages.

MISSING INFORMATION

Information is missing from routinely collected clinical data; Sod's law usually means that it is just the data you need that are missing. Dinesh faces exactly that problem.

Dinesh

Dinesh's procedure for data collection is fairly typical of situations where the researcher collects data from routine health service information that has already been gathered in the course of clinical practice. The trouble with routine clinical data is that many potentially useful characteristics of patients, or of the care they receive, are not recorded consistently. For example, he wanted to know whether patients who had self-harmed had attended on their own or were accompanied by a friend or relative – because it is relevant to the question of whether advocacy might be valuable or not. He therefore included this item on the research project's data collection sheet. Unfortunately, in the event, this detail proved to be missing from the great majority of case records. Inaccuracy and missing values thereby made it impossible for him to examine whether being accompanied or not was related to care received and arrangements made for discharge and aftercare. Because he planned to meet directly with a sample of patients, to ask about their interest in an advocacy service, he realised that he would be able to ask at that point about whether they were accompanied and, for this subgroup of the whole sample, he would be able to record information on this variable.

There are a couple of reasons why it might be worth recording information about being accompanied to the ED despite frequent occurrence of missing values. First, Dinesh might have been planning a qualitative component to the study. If so, recording for some patients the presence of an accompanying person would have been useful for purposive sampling, even though the information was usually missing (see Chapter 8). Second (probably not applicable here), there are some items of information that ought to be collected by a clinical service when dealing with patients. It can be of interest in research (or audit) that some important particular is frequently missing from the record. Where the information is necessary for a satisfactory clinical assessment, it will often be reasonable to conclude that the lack of a record means that the assessment itself was incomplete. The missing item can thereby become part of the analysis and lead to suggestions for improved clinical assessment.

Dinesh's draft data sheet

Dinesh asks his supervisor, who has experience of this kind of thing, for an opinion about his data collection sheet. She thinks it is good work. It allows for one person reattending and thereby being responsible for more than one episode. It codes the data in a way that will readily feed into data analysis software such as SPSS, which they plan to use. The way he proposes to collect the data is in a format recognised by SPSS. Where appropriate he has included codes for missing data when the ED record simply doesn't contain the information. For the recording of level of consciousness, his codes accommodate the exact entry of Glasgow Coma Scale (GCS) values if they are set out in the case notes, and he has allowed for entry of an estimated category if GCS scores are not described; the GCS scores can be converted to the four broad categories in the analysis. She thinks that the codes for the drugs taken are probably too numerous, being sceptical whether this much detail is needed for the answering of Dinesh's main study questions. On the other hand, she points out to him that he will probably want to record some simple subcategories of injury such as cutting, burning, jumping, and other methods of injury.

PRIMARY USE OF COMPUTERS FOR COLLECTING AND CODING

In some large research projects, data coding is streamlined by creating and printing special coding sheets that are filled in by hand but can then be read by an optical scanner directly into computer software. This can be a huge time-saver when the quantity of data is large, but the use of these techniques is not a simple matter. There are equipment costs and software costs but, most especially, we have found that the expertise in the initial setting up of the coding sheets can be the biggest stumbling block. We would not recommend optical scanning procedures outside of a substantial and well-funded research project – one in which there is the funding for bespoke design of the coding sheets by an expert. We have found that local expertise in the use of optical scanning for administrative activities doesn't translate to expertise in research. Beware!

We (the authors) are of a certain age (for example, we think it unlikely that any of us will ever switch from print media to eBooks and electronic readers). Bearing in mind our Luddite tendencies, it is our opinion that coding data on to paper still holds attractions for researchers, and especially so in smaller projects where the design for the coding is your own or that of your small team of colleagues. The situation is quite different when, in a larger project, coding databases for laptop or handheld computers can be commissioned by you from experts in the field of data collection.

SECURITY

Despite the misgivings expressed above, many researchers successfully use portable computers to collect and code their data in one step instead of collecting on paper and transferring to computer later. If this is the case, there are some things to remember.

Computers are expensive and attractive to thieves. It is disastrous if confidential data are lost – as they may be if a portable computer is left unattended or snatched. Consequently, very great care must be taken over the anonymity of data held on computers, and encryption of various kinds will often be required. Of course, paper files can be lost too but they are less alluring to potential thieves, and less vulnerable when the researcher is on the move (because the data collected earlier are usually back in the office). Remember also that laptop computers can be surprisingly heavy and bulky; lugging heavy equipment around hospitals and clinics can be detrimental to the researcher's musculoskeletal system (usually adversely affecting the back and neck).

There are some useful ways of protecting identifying data, whether on computer or paper. If possible, complete anonymisation can be undertaken when the data are collected. It might, for example, be unnecessary ever to record the identity, or potential identifiers such as date of birth or address, of the subjects of a study using routinely collected data. If that is the case, there is a much reduced security concern about the project. All too often, though, it is important to be able to determine who is a subject or participant – for example, when multiple episodes of care need to be assigned to a single person. Under these circumstances, there are various ways of hiding the identity in a secure way.

Lists that contain real identifying data (names, dates of birth, addresses, postcodes, hospital numbers, and the like) can be held entirely separately from other lists whose only identifier is unique to the project. This second list can contain the clinical variables that have been coded up; if it were lost or stolen there could be no identification of a person from any of the clinical data because the other list would be needed for this step – and it is held elsewhere. If the list of names and other identifying data is lost, there are no clinical details alongside the 'names'. With such a system the two lists are never alongside one another except back in the secure setting of the office and, most especially, never both in transit or in a busy clinical area together. Keeping the lists apart means never holding them on the same portable hard drive or data stick, even when the data are encrypted. There is much to be said for not holding any data on a portable computer's hard drive. Data sticks can be safer provided that the data are coded on the portable machine straight to the stick, encrypted there, and never brought together on the portable computer with the true identifying variables.

In the office too there need to be strict procedures for data protection. Computers in the office need security measures, for switching on and logging in, but also for what might be visible to other office users. There need to be locked cabinets or drawers for papers that record confidential material. Rooms may need to be locked when not occupied by researchers and the installation of door keypads is sometimes appropriate within research or healthcare buildings. There should usually be arrangements with senior colleagues to cover the possibility that the principal investigator might be unavailable, so that the data cannot be lost or beyond access because of prolonged absence of the principal researcher. Ethics and governance demand that data, once collected, should be put to the purpose intended.

In some circumstances there may need to be access, when required, to an approved person from whichever department in the research's host organisation deals with research governance. Your procedures should be able to stand up to this reasonable scrutiny on behalf of the patients and healthcare organisations that have supplied the data.

DATA COLLECTION DIRECTLY FROM THE STUDY PARTICIPANT

So far in this chapter the assumption has been that the data for the study are being extracted from existing records, registers, case notes and the like. Often, however, researchers will meet directly with the participants in the research, and the study data will be generated by way of a conversation with the patient or client. There are many similarities between direct contact and extraction of data from records. Particularly common is the categorisation and coding of likely responses, with the intention of analysing these data on the computer in a quantitative way. Qualitative approaches to data collection are dealt with in Chapter 12.

If data are to be collected directly from the patient, the place of the meeting is one of the first things to arrange once the matter of consent (Chapter 16) has been sorted out. There are many possibilities, all of which are widely used in health research. Research interviews take place in clinics and wards – either while study participants are already there for a clinical reason, or during visits that have been specially arranged for the purpose of the research. In other projects, the interviews occur at the patient's home.

There are many and varied considerations. Safety is crucial and particular care is needed concerning researchers' visits to patients' homes, and for meetings that may be in quiet and lonely clinic rooms; research interviews not uncommonly take place outside of the normal working day, for the convenience of the participant who may be in employment and sparing their time out of normal working hours. The procedures for safety are largely those of clinical practice itself. In particular, whether the interviewer has prior knowledge of the person is important, as is the nature of the topic being studied; plainly, a sample of patients who have severe renal disease or have had a stroke pose different safety implications from samples where the patients consume excessive alcohol or have walked out of a care setting before their care was completed. Visits to people's homes need a clear protocol for the visit, which should be worked out with colleagues experienced in such work. Arrangements will take account of any accompanying person, expected duration of the trip, arrangements for reporting in once back at base, and so on. The host institution for the research ought to have in place guidelines or, better, clear procedures for clinical and research visits.

Some quantitative projects will require measurement of the repeatability of interviews – most often measurement of inter-rater repeatability (or inter-rater reliability). This might involve someone else listening to an audio (or less often a video) recording of a sample of the interviews, and rating the participant's responses on the questionnaire – to see whether they get the same ratings as you did.

In qualitative research, it is standard practice for one-to-one interviews to be audio-recorded; the transcriptions of the recordings form the data of the study and the basis of the analysis. Consent for such recordings is dealt with in Chapter 16. It can't be stressed too strongly that equipment should be tested and you should be familiar with it before setting it up in the presence of the study participant. With technology, if things can go wrong they will. Generally speaking, if an hour-long recorded interview turns out not to be recorded because of technical failure (often human error) it won't be possible to go back another time and do the whole thing again. One chance.

Getting the equipment right is part of a wider arrangement for the interview. Often you will plan to use a topic guide or a questionnaire (or a number of questionnaires). The paper version of these documents needs to be in a format that you find usable. Your questions must flow from one item to the next, and your practice with the documents to hand should ensure that you can conduct the interview in an efficient and professional way. This may mean a fair bit of work on the format of the paper documents before you get around to practising the interview with a colleague. People differ in their liking for folders, staples, single or double-sided paper, treasury tags to hold sheets together, and flash cards (used when asking participants to select appropriate responses from lists of items). You should get the package ready in the way that suits your personal style.

Remember that you are often on something of a race against time. Participants will only take part for a limited time, and you may be trying to squeeze in a lot of data collecting during that short period. In some studies it will be reasonable to return on another occasion if the work is unfinished. This should be

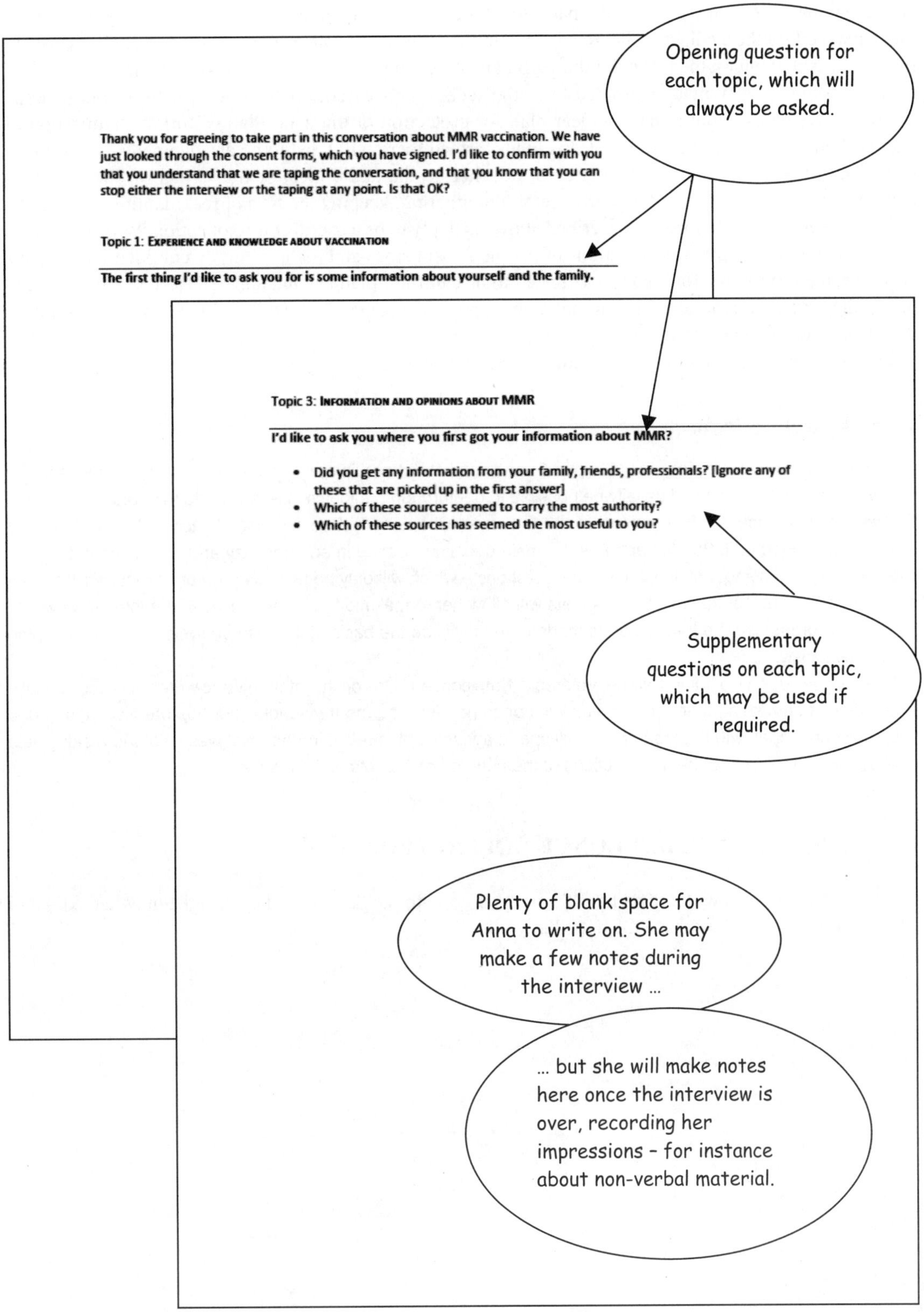

Opening question for each topic, which will always be asked.

Thank you for agreeing to take part in this conversation about MMR vaccination. We have just looked through the consent forms, which you have signed. I'd like to confirm with you that you understand that we are taping the conversation, and that you know that you can stop either the interview or the taping at any point. Is that OK?

Topic 1: EXPERIENCE AND KNOWLEDGE ABOUT VACCINATION

The first thing I'd like to ask you for is some information about yourself and the family.

Topic 3: INFORMATION AND OPINIONS ABOUT MMR

I'd like to ask you where you first got your information about MMR?

- Did you get any information from your family, friends, professionals? [Ignore any of these that are picked up in the first answer]
- Which of these sources seemed to carry the most authority?
- Which of these sources has seemed the most useful to you?

Supplementary questions on each topic, which may be used if required.

Plenty of blank space for Anna to write on. She may make a few notes during the interview …

… but she will make notes here once the interview is over, recording her impressions – for instance about non-verbal material.

FIGURE 18.2 Draft pages from Anna's semi-structured interview schedule.

an exceptional step, at the grace of the participant, rather than a regular occurrence because you have too much planned for the available time. Research interviewing can be rather like packing for a holiday, where the advice is: lay out on the bed everything you absolutely must take, and then take only half of it.

As with the security matters alluded to in the section above about data collection from routine data, it will always be essential to have a clear plan for protection of the data. Plainly, full anonymisation of data will not be possible in a study of this kind. Instead there will need to be arrangements for ensuring that identifying names and numbers are not attached to the audio-files, or transcripts of interviews, or any other materials. Some kind of study identity numbering, keeping the lists of real identifiers and study identifiers separate at all times, as described above, is likely to be a useful course of action. With audio-files and transcripts where there are mentions of people's real names and perhaps highly confidential narrative accounts, the procedures for security will need to be carefully planned and adhered to. There will need to be a policy for destruction of the material at an appropriate stage in the study – local ethical committees will usually offer advice on the timing of such procedures.

Let's see how Anna is progressing with her data collection.

Anna's data collection

Anna has discussed her topic guide (Chapter 9) and semi-structured interview schedule with her supervisor and they have agreed that it should usually be possible to get through the topics in less than 45 minutes. She has set out for herself on paper the four topics that she will cover (Chapter 14). She has placed each of the four topics on a single page (Figure 18.2). First appears the main question, framed in an open way and which she will always ask, followed by a number of supplementary questions – which will only be used as prompts if required. The rest of the space on each of the four single sheets will allow her to make jotted notes. Because the interviews will all be audio-recorded and the transcriptions made of them will be the basis of the data analysis, she does not plan to write copiously.

She and her supervisor think it will be preferable if she concentrates on the interview and writes only occasionally when there is something that she believes will not stand alone on the transcript. After the interview has ended and she is no longer with the mother she will spend a few minutes reflecting on what was said and making field notes, topic by topic, about her recollections of the non-verbal aspects of the interview.

DEALING WITH THE DATA ONCE COLLECTED

The next chapter deals with the matter of what you do with the data once they have been collected – and what to do when you don't have the data that you want.

19

Living With (and Without) the Data

QUANTITATIVE DATA AND THE COMPUTER

Data will usually need to be entered (typed) into the computer so that they can be analysed using a designated research data software application such as SPSS. One of the simplest ways to transfer data to a computer file from the coding sheet that you used in the fieldwork is to use, first of all, a readily available application such as Microsoft's Word or Excel or Notepad. Type all of the numbers or alphabetical characters coded on each participant's (or subject's) coding sheet into a single row (*rows* are horizontal while *columns* are vertical). The numbers need to be spaced so that each variable – age, sex, medicine taken, and so on – is separated from the preceding and successive variable. The Tab key is probably the best separator to use. In Figure 19.1 you will see an extract showing the kind of data that Dinesh collected and the way that the numbers form the first line of the Word document he created.

Notice that the first number of every line is the unique identifying number for each episode. In this study *episodes* are the unit of assessment in the sample; more often, *participants* form the units – but here, one patient may be responsible for more than one episode. In every study there must be a unique identifier for the unit of assessment. Because each row of data has its unique identifying number, you can sort the file by any other variable and still locate exactly which episode (or more usually, person) the other variables refer to.

When this task is done, all of the data on the original coding sheets used in the fieldwork have been represented, line by line and episode by episode, on the Word document. Next comes the important step of saving this data file in a format that can be recognised by SPSS (or other statistical application). The usual format for the saving of a word-processed file may not work well with the chosen statistical application. These data files should be saved in a more rudimentary format such as Plain Text, where various fancy features of the word processor are pared down to the bone. Some people favour typing data into Notepad, the exceptionally basic text editor offered with all common versions of Microsoft Windows (accessed through the package of features to be found in the 'Accessories' folder among 'All Programs'). Alternatively you might prefer to use the spreadsheet function of Excel, placing each variable into a different cell.

SPSS itself has a data entry feature and it offers a spreadsheet into which data can be typed directly. We prefer to compile a data file and then feed that file into SPSS The statistical applications such as SPSS recognise the common types of data file and import the data effectively from a Word or Excel file.

A short instruction course (a few hours) in the use of SPSS or Minitab teaches how to import the data, sort out special sorts of variables such as dates and times of day, label the variables, define the values of each variable (e.g. 1 = male, 2 = female), and sort out the missing data values. This last point is important. You should notice that there must be some value typed in for every variable for every person in the study.

Getting Started in Health Research, First Edition. David Bowers, Allan House and David Owens.
© 2011 David Bowers, Allan House and David Owens. Published 2011 by Blackwell Publishing Ltd.

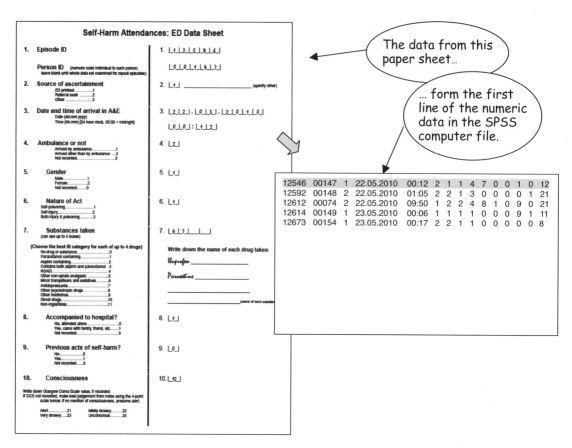

FIGURE 19.1   Dinesh's coding sheet converted to a computer file.

If there were missing items, the order of variables across the rows would vary from one person to another and the resulting columns would not represent the data correctly. The example in Figure 19.1 shows the use of missing values to prevent such a mishap, ensuring that the data for every one of the five people shown is set out in 15 columns, where each column represents the correct values coded for that variable.

The picture in Figure 19.2 shows how the same five people's data are displayed in SPSS once the data file has been imported and the variables have been given their appropriate labels: sex, age and so on. Figure 19.3 shows exactly the same data with one refinement: the values for each variable have been labelled in SPSS, so that their meaning can be shown whenever any analysis is undertaken (Chapter 21). This book will not take further the matter of how data are analysed in SPSS; this kind of tuition is available, formally and informally. Many people find the analysis itself a satisfying, straightforward and even enjoyable task, and one that is easily learned to a basic level of competence.

REFUSALS TO PARTICIPATE, DROP-OUTS AND OTHER MISSING PERSONS

Some people will decline an invitation to take part in research and, in studies based on case records, some records won't be found and subjects consequently not included. Deciding what to do in these circumstances is challenging. No hard and fast rules apply. Pilot and feasibility work will help you avoid

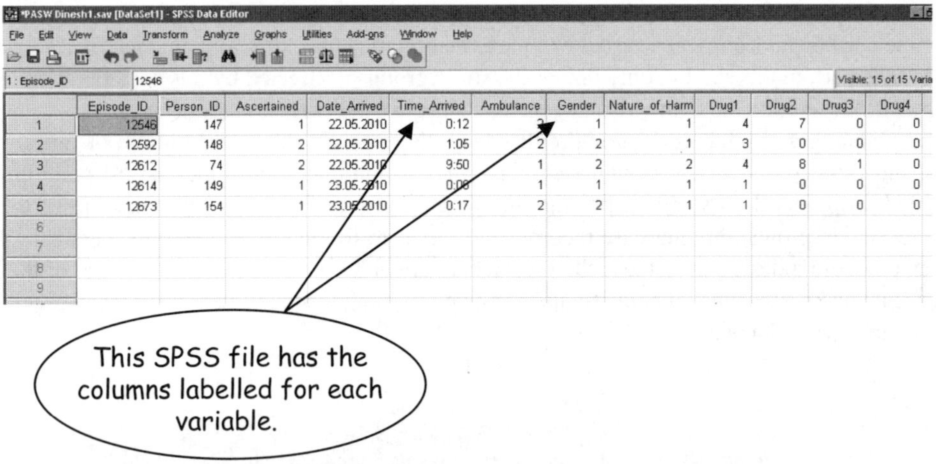

FIGURE 19.2   Dinesh's data – an extract from the SPSS file.

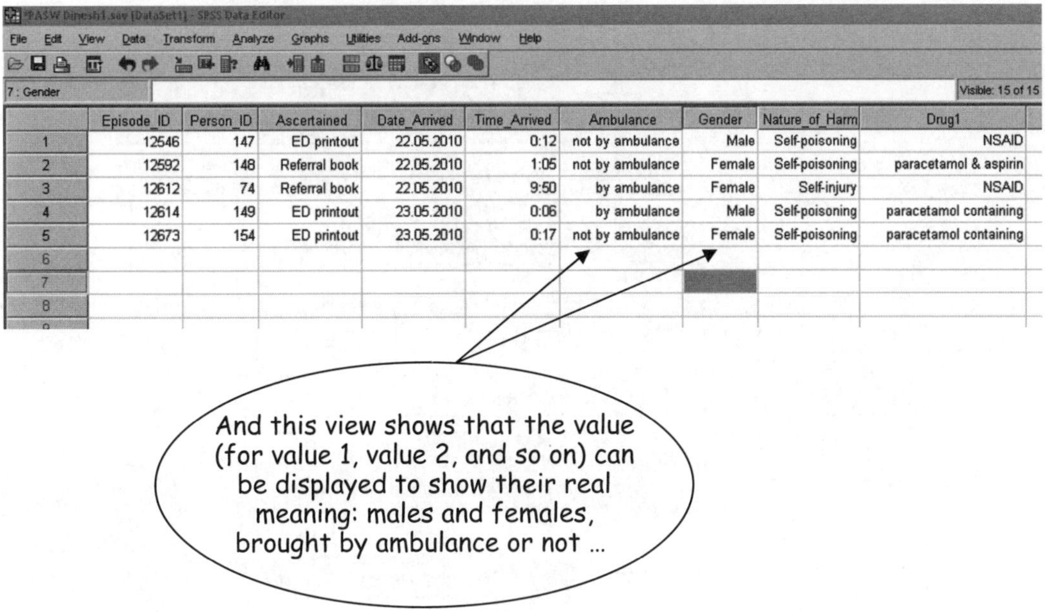

FIGURE 19.3   Dinesh's data – an extract of the SPSS file, showing value labels.

problems like these. Refusals and missing inclusions aren't usually a devastating flaw in a study unless they are numerous.

Exclusions and drop-outs from studies have effects that depend on many factors – but the study's design is especially important. In a randomised controlled trial, people who don't take part affect the extent to which the findings can be generalised to the target population, but those included are randomly assigned to one or other treatment; the non-participation doesn't introduce a between-group bias. But in the selection of participants in a case-control study, it is quite possible that the 'cases', being people affected by the condition, may be enthusiastic about taking part – in the hope of contributing to useful knowledge about their condition. Controls, unaffected by the condition being studied, have less at stake and some may decline enrolment. Those who turn down participation may have different characteristics from those willing to take part; in this setting, only one of the study groups is affected by this consideration, and bias is thereby introduced into the comparison of the exposures of the cases and the controls.

Careful planning and pilot work should either keep these problems to a minimum or reveal a major flaw that must be tackled in the design stage. The next important step is the careful recording of all refusals and drop-outs. It is standard practice in clinical trials to provide a flow diagram of the whole study: refusals, drop-outs, missing case records, and losses to follow up (see below). Figure 19.4 is one such example from a descriptive study; the researchers are able to provide a clear picture of the study's strengths and weaknesses when it came to including and keeping the participants that were targeted when the investigation was planned.

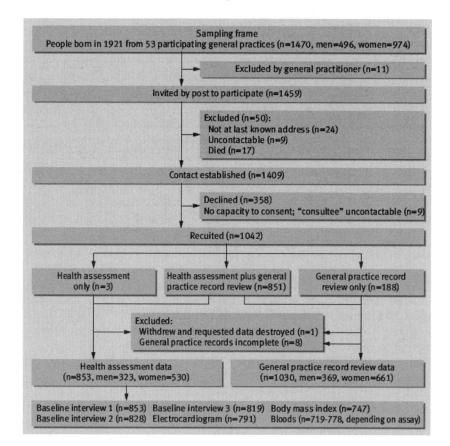

FIGURE 19.4 A flow diagram from a cohort analytic study.

MISSING A LOT OF DATA

Sadly, we sometimes have more data missing than just a few values for a few variables, as in the example earlier. Of course the researcher does his or her best to keep such loss to a minimum because it badly disrupts the analysis and may, in the end, raise doubts about the findings. But research is a real-world activity and there will sometimes be unavoidable losses of data; how are these events to be tackled?

One of the decisions to be made concerns the rules for collection. For example, if there is to be a follow-up collection of data at six months, what if the due date is missed (perhaps the patient was out of town, or the researcher poorly)? Will it be acceptable to include data taken at seven months (or if an absence was predicted, perhaps at five months)? The basic answer, as with so many things, is to set out the rules in advance. Of course there is a time that is so distant from the intended date that it is ridiculous to include data from that point with the properly collected data for everyone else in the study. But what is the acceptable window of time? There is no correct answer save that of deciding what is reasonable, what can be sensibly written into the final report, and sticking to it. That period might be six months, give or take two weeks, or perhaps within one month either side of the due date. The big worry is that, at the end of a comparison study, one of the groups being compared will have been followed up sooner than the other. If the researchers are doing their job properly, the small discrepancies should be randomly distributed between the two groups and there will be little likelihood of any important bias.

It is regarded as good practice in clinical trials for all participants who were randomly allocated to be accounted for in the final analysis of data concerning the main outcomes. The corollary is that it is unacceptable for patients who drop out to be disregarded in the analysis. This seemingly rather odd rule is known as 'Intention-to-Treat Analysis' (ITT) and has become adopted as standard procedure. The reason is that there is good evidence that ITT diminishes the biases that are introduced by people who drop out of a trial after having been randomly allocated to one or other treatment. One problem that it introduces, however, is the conundrum of what to do when analysing the outcome data when the data for some participants are missing because they have dropped out of follow-up. To deal with the missing data researchers sometimes use a procedure known as 'Last Observation Carried Forwards' (LOCF). Basically this step assumes that the last available data remain constant over the time not accounted for because of the loss of contact. This will often be a conservative estimate of any treatment effect, but its effects on the final trial analysis are unpredictable and no one is very happy about its use; it is widely regarded as an attempt to make the best of a bad job.

Statisticians have in recent years made considerable advances in the study of missing data. In certain circumstances, usually in large studies, they are able to create mathematical models in which missing data can be (apparently) reliably imputed (or made up).

The main point to be made is that missing follow-up data cannot merely be disregarded, while the necessary attempts that researchers make to deal with the absence are complex, flawed, unsatisfactory, and awkward to explain in the write-up. The failure to capture the expected data in any appreciable volume is bad news for the research.

QUALITATIVE RESEARCH AND MISSING DATA

As with quantitative research, all too often the written account of a qualitative study fails to set out sufficient information about the sample and, in particular, doesn't say enough about who refused to take part or dropped out. This information is part of a qualitative study's methods and results, and it should be summarised. Sometimes, in a purposive sample, one or more sections of the intended sample are under-represented or missing entirely. This event is a finding of the research and should be reported – and will probably be a legitimate focus of reflection by the researcher – as to its possible reasons.

Topic guides and interview schedules are often constructed to capture particular aspects of the service users' (or carers') experiences; in the event they may fail to do so. Once again, this is important material and needs discussion. The reason may be an important one – for example, there may be avoidance of asking or responding because of some relevant aspect of the condition or its treatment.

In some but not all qualitative designs, the questions are revised repeatedly as the project continues. More often the plan for the interview or focus group is fairly fixed once the study has started. It can be extremely valuable to involve (to employ) service users as interviewers in qualitative studies because they may stand the best chance of eliciting the relevant data despite these potential impediments. Of course, regardless of who will be carrying out the interviews or focus groups, careful consultation with service users beforehand will be invaluable – as will sufficient pilot work before embarking on the project proper. We haven't set out any of Dinesh's plans for the small qualitative component of his study. He plans to ask a sample of the patients who have self-harmed about their views concerning advocacy – were it to become available in a clinical trial. If he is to get any meaningful findings in his study he would do well, before he begins interviewing, to check carefully with some service users whether they have any idea what he means by advocacy; we (the authors) have some experience that suggests that he will have to work hard to explain to his participants what the concept might mean in practice.

VI

Staying the Course

20

Taking Stock

A PROGRESS REPORT

It might be useful to review where you've got to so far. You've:

- Defined your research question in detail – you know exactly what you want to do (Chapter 1);
- Done a preliminary search of the existing literature, and had a quick look at what's out there. You didn't find anything obvious that you need to worry about (Chapter 2);
- Written a draft plan of your research – what you will do and how you will do it (Chapter 3);
- Done a thorough literature search. You're satisfied that you are not about to duplicate someone else's work (Chapter 4);
- Thought about who can help you in your research: a supervisor or mentor; a clinical collaborator; other professionals (perhaps, for example, a statistician or an information specialist); perhaps a service user (Chapter 5);
- Decided on an appropriate study design. If quantitative then a cross-sectional study, a case-control study, a trial, and so on. If qualitative then possibly a purposive design (Chapter 6);
- Decided on your sample. Which sampling procedure? How you will select the participants? Who will be included (and who will be excluded)? (Chapter 7 for the quantitative case, Chapter 8 for the qualitative case);
- Looked at what information you want to collect from each of your research subjects (Chapter 9);
- Thought about the problem of confounders if your research is quantitative (Chapter 10);
- Decided how many subjects you need to include in your sample (Chapter 11);
- Got yourself ready to do the research, including a decision as to what method of analysis you will apply to your data. What things will you need to set in place? What special knowledge (e.g. data analysis software or statistical methods) will you need? (Chapter 12 for the qualitative research case, Chapter 13 for the quantitative case);
- Written your definitive research protocol (Chapter 14);
- Made sure that you have any necessary funding in place (Chapter 15);
- Got any necessary permissions or approvals for your research – ethical, NHS, etc. (Chapter 16);
- Considered the practicalities of approaching and recruiting your research subjects (Chapter 17);
- Decided how you are going to collect and record the data – data collection forms, coding, questionnaires, using computers (Chapter 18);
- Thought about how you will deal with any missing data (Chapter 19).

The remaining chapters of the book deal with the processes involved in dealing with the results and the outcomes of research. From now on we won't be making any detailed references to Dinesh and Anna, whose work (and existence) was fictitious, although we may allude to them occasionally. Their projects can carry on largely without us looking over their shoulders.

Getting Started in Health Research, First Edition. David Bowers, Allan House and David Owens.
© 2011 David Bowers, Allan House and David Owens. Published 2011 by Blackwell Publishing Ltd.

21

Making Sense of Your Results – the Quantitative Case

INTRODUCTION

Now that you've got some quantitative data, you can apply the method of analysis you chose in Chapter 13, and begin to throw some light on your research question. Regardless of what more complex methods of analysis you intend to use, you will generally want to start with a table of basic characteristics, or baseline table, which tells the reader about the subjects you've been working with. This table is an essential feature of any written research results.

Usually these tables will contain some demographic data (age, sex, ethnicity, occupation, etc.), along with information particularly relevant to the study in question, for example duration and severity of current illness, previous clinical history, and so on. To summarise these data and describe the distribution of the variables you can use:

- percentages or proportions (for example, to indicate the relative proportions of males and females in the sample);
- means and standard deviations (if your data are metric);
- or medians and interquartile ranges (if your data are ordinal or skewed metric).

Although we can't show you Dinesh's results because he only exists in our imagination, here are some results from similar papers.

Figure 21.1 is an example of a simple baseline table and is taken from a study of salbutamol in asthma control. Baseline tables don't come much more basic than this; it shows some demographic data and some study-relevant clinical data.

A somewhat more complicated baseline table is shown in Figure 21.2, taken from a randomised double-blind placebo-controlled trial of nitazoxanide for the treatment of severe rotavirus diarrhoea. This table, as well as showing the basic characteristics of the subjects in both groups (active suspension versus the placebo) also compares the values in each category (see the 'p-values' in the last column). Note that we have truncated the table a little to save space.

Dinesh will want to construct a baseline table describing the subjects in his study – and so will you.

Getting Started in Health Research, First Edition. David Bowers, Allan House and David Owens.

Regular vs as-needed inhaled salbutamol in asthma control

Kenneth R Chapman, Steven Kesten, John Paul Szalal

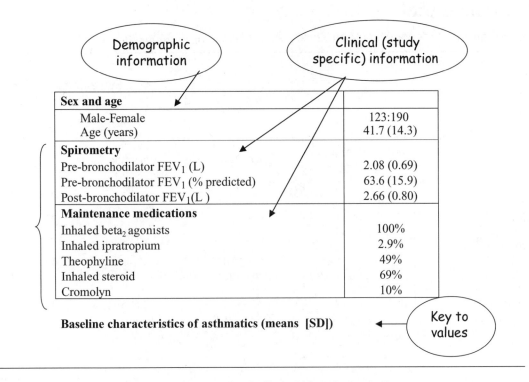

FIGURE 21.1   A simple baseline table from a study of salbutamol in asthma control.

AFTER THE TABLE OF BASIC CHARACTERISTICS – WHAT NEXT?

The baseline table describes the principal features of the sample subjects. You will follow this by presenting your main results. You might want to start simply, perhaps with a chart (for example, a bar chart, boxplot, or histogram), or with a frequency table. A chart is useful if you want to explain something which would be difficult to explain easily with either a table or with text. After this, your results can become progressively more complex – you want essentially to lead your readers by the hand. An example of a clustered bar chart is shown in Figure 21.3, and a histogram in Figure 21.4. You might also want to provide a flow chart to provide a visual account of the whole study process (numbers recruited, excluded, drop-outs, losses to follow-up, and so on) – see Chapters 17 and 19 for more on these.

As for tables displaying results, you will almost certainly need to use more than one. Once again start with the simpler table, and progress to more complex layouts as you work through your results. For example, Figure 21.5 is a simple frequency table showing adverse events in 60 participants with migraine treated with either lisinopril or placebo.

Figure 21.6 is a more complex table from the same study and compares primary outcomes using confidence intervals. Notice the desirable use of the word 'to' in the confidence interval rather than a comma or a hyphen.

Effect of nitazoxanide for the treatment of severe rotavirus diarrhea: randomised double-blind placebo-controlled trial

Jean-Francois Rosignol, Mona Abu-Zeckry, Abeer Hussain, M Gabriella Santoro

> Some demographic variables ...

	All patients	Active suspension	Placebo suspension	P*
Race				
White	38	18	20	1.0
Sex				
Male	21	9	12	0.75
Female	17	9	8	
Age (months)				
Mean (SD)	15.1 (15.5)	16.9 (22.1)	13.4 (4.9)	0.52
Median (range)	11.0 (5-92)	9.0 (5-92)	12.0 (5-24)	
Weight				
Mean (SD)	8.2 (2.6)	8.2 (3.6)	8.2 (1.5)	0.93
Median (range)	7.8 (5.0-20.0)	7.2 (5.0-20.0)	8.3 (6.1-11.4)	
Stool frequency				
3-4/day	5	4	1	0.27
5-10/day	26	11	15	
>10/day	7	3	4	
Stool consistency				
Liquid	38	18	20	1.0
Vomiting				
Yes	30	13	17	0.44
No	8	5	3	
Malnutrition status				
Severely underweight	11	5	6	0.95
Moderately underweight	11	6	5	
Mildly underweight	9	4	5	
Not underweight	7	3	4	

Fisher's exact test or x^2 test used for comparing proportions, t-test for means.

> ... and some clinical, study-related, variables.

FIGURE 21.2 A table of baseline characteristics taken from a randomised double-blind placebo-controlled trial of nitazoxanide for the treatment of severe rotavirus diarrhoea. This table shows the basic characteristics of the subjects in both groups (active suspension versus the placebo).

Newly diagnosed idiopathic thrombocytopenic purpura in childhood: an observational study

Thomas Kühne, Paul Imbach, Paula H B Bolton-Maggs, Willi Berchtold, Victor Blanchette, George R Buchanan, for the Intercontinental Childhood ITP Study Group

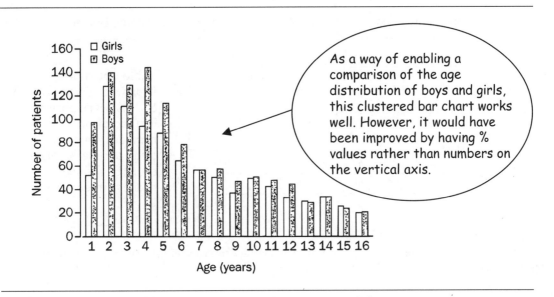

FIGURE 21.3 A clustered bar chart showing the age distribution by gender of a sample of children with idiopathic thrombocytopenic purpura (ITP).

Serum Potassium, Cigarette Smoking, and Mortality in Middle-aged Men

S. Goya Wannamethee[1], Anthony F. Lever[2], A. Gerald Shaper[1] and Peter H. Whincup[1]

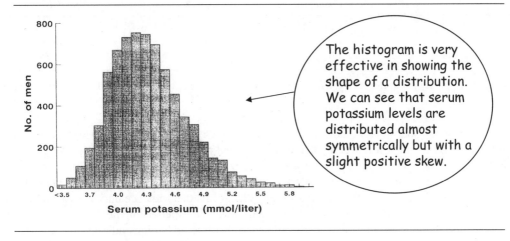

FIGURE 21.4 A histogram of serum potassium levels in 7262 middle-aged men who were not receiving treatment for hypertension. British Regional Heart Study, 1978–1991.

Prophylactic treatment of migraine with angiotensin converting enzyme inhibitor (lisinopril): randomised, placebo controlled, crossover study

Harald Schrader, Lars Jacob Stovner, Grethe Helde, Trond Sand, Gunnar Bovim

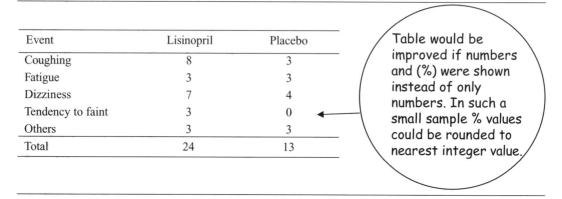

Event	Lisinopril	Placebo
Coughing	8	3
Fatigue	3	3
Dizziness	7	4
Tendency to faint	3	0
Others	3	3
Total	24	13

Table would be improved if numbers and (%) were shown instead of only numbers. In such a small sample % values could be rounded to nearest integer value.

FIGURE 21.5   Adverse events in 60 participants with migraine treated with lisinopril or placebo (note: only 47 patients actually evaluated due to drop-outs for various reasons).

Prophylactic treatment of migraine with angiotensin converting enzyme inhibitor (lisinopril): randomised, placebo controlled, crossover study

Harald Schrader, Lars Jacob Stovner, Grethe Helde, Trond Sand, Gunnar Bovim

Primary efficacy parameter	Lisinopril	Placebo	Mean % reduction (95% CI)
Hours with headache	129 (125)	162 (142)	20 (5 to 36)
Days with headache	19.7 (14)	23.7 (11)	17 (5 to 30)
Days with migraine	14.5 (11)	18.5 (10)	21 (9 to 34)

FIGURE 21.6   Efficacy parameters in 47 participants with migraine during treatment periods of 12 weeks. Figures are means (SD).

If you are presenting odds, risk or hazard ratios, or regression results, you might want to consider starting with unadjusted results first, followed by the results adjusted for confounders and so on. As a reminder, unadjusted results are those which take no account of the influence of other potentially confounding variables on the relationship in question (we first introduced the idea of confounders in Chapter 10).

As an example, Figure 21.7 is from a study of the effect of partner violence during pregnancy, on the odds of women having postnatal depression, compared to women experiencing no partner violence. The table shows first the unadjusted (crude) odds ratios and then the odds ratios adjusted for a number of potentially confounding variables (see table footnote for the variables adjusted for) (note: table slightly truncated).

Violence against women by their intimate partner during pregnancy and postnatal depression: a prospective cohort study

Ana Bernado Ludermir, Glyn Lewis, Sandra Alves Valonguiero, Thalia Velho Barreto de Arauja, Ricardo Araya

	Total participants (n = 1045)	Total participants with postnatal depression (n = 270)*	Unadjusted odds ratio (95% CI)‡	Adjusted odds ratio (95% CI)
None	724 (69%)	131 (18%)	1.00	1.00
Physical or sexual violence alone	27 (3%)	7 (26%)	1.58 (0.65–3.82)	1.03 (0.40–2.64)
Psychological violence alone	174 (17%)	68 (39%)	2.90 (2.03–4.16)	2.13 (1.45–3.13)
Physical or sexual violence plus psychological violence	120 (11%)	64 (53%)	5.17 (3.45–7.76)	2.83 (1.76–4.55)
p values			<0.0001	<0.0001

SRQ-20 self-reporting questionnaire with 20 items. * Percentages are the proportion of the total number of participants who have experienced each type of violence. ‡ Adjusted for age, race, marital status, years of schooling, employment status, communication with present or most recent partner, controlling behaviour of present or most recent partner, social support, and length of follow-up.

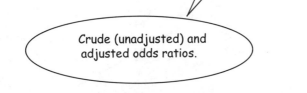

Crude (unadjusted) and adjusted odds ratios.

FIGURE 21.7   Crude and adjusted odds ratios (and 95%CI) of having postnatal depression with different levels of exposure to partner violence during pregnancy, compared to women experiencing no partner violence.

RE-VISITING THE CONFOUNDING PROBLEM – STRATIFICATION AND MODELLING

When we first mentioned confounding in Chapter 10, we said that it can be dealt with either at the design stage or at the analysis stage. There are two principal ways of dealing with confounders during the analysis stage – either with stratification methods, or by modelling, that is, using regression methods. With the stratification approach (as we noted in Chapter 10) you need to identify relevant strata *before* you collect the data, and then ensure that you have enough subjects in each stratum (using a power calculation if necessary).

For example, researchers who compared patterns of hospital care and repetition associated with self-poisoning and self-injury (including cutting), were interested in the proportion of patients who received a psychosocial assessment. They found a 'striking association' between the method of self-harm used and whether the person received a psychosocial assessment. The authors compared receipt of a psychosocial assessment among the self-cutting-only group with receipt of assessment among all other methods of self-harm and found an odds ratio of 0.35, with a 95% CI of (0.30–0.40). Since psychosocial assessment is more likely after admission to the general hospital than it is after discharge directly from the emergency department, the authors adjusted the above odds ratios with a stratified analysis for the confounding effects of hospital admission. This confirmed that there is a clear relationship between self-cutting and a failure to receive psychosocial assessment that is not explained by admission to the general hospital – adjusted OR = 0.64, 95% CI (0.54–0.75). These results are shown in Figure 21.8.

Hospital care and repetition following self-harm: multicentre comparison of self-poisoning and self-injury

Rachael Lilley, David Owens, Judith Horrocks, Allan House, Rachael Noble *et al.*

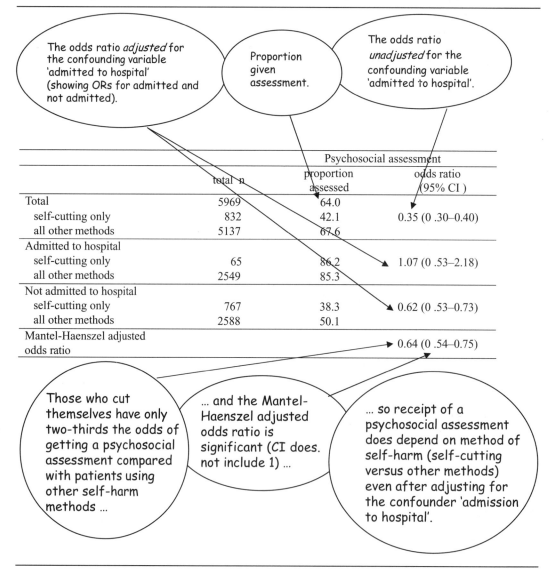

FIGURE 21.8   The odds ratio of a patient receiving a psychosocial assessment after self-harm, according to whether the method of harm was self-cutting only, adjusting for whether admitted to hospital or not.

You can combine the odds ratios using the Mantel-Haenszel procedure and test the hypothesis that the method of self-harm and receiving psychosocial assessment are independent when stratified by the confounder hospital admission. The combined odds ratio of 0.64 (which is significant since the confidence interval does not include 1) shows that these are not independent. If you are not already familiar with this procedure you will need to get some statistical advice.

The stratification method of dealing with confounders and the accompanying Mantel-Haenszel test is appropriate if the variables are categorical (or can be made so), and if there is only *one* confounder, but otherwise can become cumbersome. With continuous variables and *more* than one possible confounder, the modelling approach, using either a linear or logistic regression equation, is preferable. In these circumstances, the primary outcome variable is placed on the left-hand side of the equation, and the favoured explanatory variable, together with any number of confounders (subject to sample size limitations), included on the right-hand side. Regression methods are easy to apply (using SPSS, Minitab or STATA, for example) and with logistic models, produce odds ratios with their confidence intervals, for each variable in the model (see Figure 21.9)

Higher Survival Rates Among Younger Patients After Pediatric Intensive Care Unit Cardiac Arrests

Peter A. Meaney, Vinay M. Nadkarni, E. Francis Cook, Marcia Testa, Mark Helfaer, William Kaye, G. Luke Larkin, Robert A. Berg, for the American Heart Association National Registry of Cardiopulmonary Resuscitation Investigators

---

Multivariable logistic regression analysis was performed on factors associated with survival in the univariate analysis ($P < 0.05$) to control for patient and event variables that may confound the relationship between age category and survival (to hospital discharge).

FIGURE 21.9   A description of the modelling approach from an investigation of survival rates among younger patients after paediatric intensive care unit cardiac arrests.

There is a wide variety of tables and charts to be seen in published papers. It will be worth having a look at a few to get a feel for what might be useful for showing (and enabling the reader to make sense of) your own research results.

22

Making Sense of Your Results – the Qualitative Case

INTRODUCTION

Now that you've got some qualitative data, you can apply the method of analysis you chose in Chapter 12 to make sense of it, and hopefully answer your research question. Following the introduction and a description of the method of analysis used, the basic demographic data are usually presented as text rather than in a table (as is the case with a quantitative project). An example is shown in the extract in Figure 22.1 taken from a study into smoking and postpartum women.

Smoking and Harm-Reduction Efforts Among Postpartum Women

Mimi Nichter, Mark Nichter, Shelly Adrian, Kate Goldade, Laura Tesler, Myra Muramoto

Of the 44 women who participated in the study postpartum, 62% (n = 27) were Anglo-American, 25% (n = 11) were Mexican American, 2% (n = 1) were African American, and 11% (n = 5) were multi-ethnic. The mean age of the participants was 24 years, with a range between 18 and 43. One half of the women were married. In all, 36% (n = 16) of women were primapara; 64% (n = 28) were multipara. In terms of educational status, 34% (n = 15) had not graduated from high school. 39% (n = 17) had a high school diploma, and 27% (n = 12) had some post-high school education.

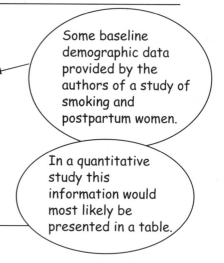

Some baseline demographic data provided by the authors of a study of smoking and postpartum women.

In a quantitative study this information would most likely be presented in a table.

FIGURE 22.1   A description of the demographic breakdown of the subjects in a qualitative study into smoking among postpartum women.

Getting Started in Health Research, First Edition. David Bowers, Allan House and David Owens.
© 2011 David Bowers, Allan House and David Owens. Published 2011 by Blackwell Publishing Ltd.

It is a good idea to provide some such demographic data to describe the background and situation of the participants in *your* study. Most qualitative papers will contain such information.

You will then want to start presenting your results. It's probably a good idea to start with a summary of your main findings (e.g. the themes identified), and then go on to elaborate and provide a more detailed explanation of what you've discovered (more details of themes, and so on). Presentation of results in qualitative research tends to be textual (and lengthy), without the use of the tables and charts found in quantitative work. Because of the (usually) lengthy description of results, it is difficult for us to provide other than sharply summarised examples of results published in journal papers. Complete examples can be found in relevant journals, for example Qualitative Health Research, which interested readers might want to consult.

Qualitative papers will often contain quotes from the participants which help to illuminate the results and findings section. For example, Figure 22.2 quotes comments made by participants in a postpartum depression study.

Women's Care-Seeking Experiences After Referral for Postpartum Depression

Wendy Sword, Dianne Busser, Rebecca Ganann, Theresa McMillan, Marilyn Swinton

---

I still don't think that what I was experiencing was postpartum depression. I think it was just an accumulation of not sleeping and being overwhelmed with the job of taking care of him. So yeah, so I'm fine with not having called anybody just because that's what I was thinking. (*Normalising of symptoms*)

I figured I did . . . I wasn't sleeping well. I was up most of the night even when the baby was asleep. I was getting really, really moody and really depressed, and really anxious and crying quite often for no really good reason. (*Symptom awareness*)

My mum and mother-in-law, they don't really understand, especially because they're kind of old world, they would just say things like, oh how can you not be happy, look at this beautiful baby, and that would just make me feel worse. (*Limited understanding by others*)

FIGURE 22.2   Comments made by participants in a qualitative study of women experiencing postpartum depression.

Anna

Anna is comfortable with the way she will cover some of these points in her written accounts, for example explaining the background to her study and the question she is asking. She can describe the interview approach she adopted and include the topic guide. She decides there are two areas where she needs to be particularly clear which research approach she took: in describing her sample; and in the approach she took to analysis of her data.

Anna decides to include basic information about her mothers with the following variables:

- Sex of index child
- Age of index child
- Number of siblings
- Vaccination history of any siblings

- Household income ($< £30$ k or $\geq £30$ k)
- Education level of mother (cessation of full-time education beyond 16, yes or no)
- Mother's age.

Anna also needs to explain how she chose the mothers to interview. She found two appropriate examples in the literature (see Figures 22.3 and 22.4). In the first, parents were selected on a number of criteria and invited to join a focus group. In the second example, the authors applied fewer selection rules but they were clearer about how they actually recruited parents.

Parents' perspectives on the MMR immunisation: a focus group study

M Evans, H Stoddart, L Condon, E Freeman, M Grizzell, and R Mullen

Six focus groups were held with parents in Avon and Gloucestershire. Three groups comprised parents who had accepted MMR for their youngest child ('immunisers') and three comprised parents who had refused MMR ('non-immunisers'). Their children had a range of histories for immunisations other than MMR. Sampling was purposeful, so that parents were included from a variety of socio-economic backgrounds who had either accepted or refused MMR immunisation for their youngest child, aged between 14 months and three years at the time of recruitment.

FIGURE 22.3   A description of the authors' subject selection procedure from a qualitative study into parents' views on MMR immunisation.

Why do parents choose not to immunise their children?

Matilda Hamilton, Paul Corwin, Suzanne Gower and Sue Rogers

Those GPs who reported to the immunisation coordinator for Pegasus Health the details of children for whom immunisation was declined (about one third of all Pegasus members) were asked to participate in this project. Parents were identified from the Pegasus Health immunisation database and their own GPs were asked to invite them to take part in the research. The lead researcher then contacted consenting parents and a face-to-face interview was arranged.

FIGURE 22.4   A description of the authors' subject selection procedure from a qualitative study of why parents do not immunise their children.

     Anna will probably model a description of her selection procedure on these two extracts. She also worried that describing her analysis might be a lengthy and intricate process given how long it took! What she discovered was that in reality most qualitative research papers simply summarise the general approach taken and refer the reader to a methodological text for details. Figure 22.5 is one example. Figure 22.6 shows another, more comprehensive, example.

     Anna also needs to think about how she will present her results, a topic to which we return in Chapter 24.

Screening and counselling for sickle cell disorders and thalassaemia: the experience of parents and health professionals

Karl Atkin, Waqar I.U. Ahmad and Elizabeth N. Anionwu

All interviews were tape-recorded. Those in Asian languages were interpreted into English. Transcribed interviews were organised according to analytical headings. Following accepted conventions of qualitative analysis (Gubrium and Silverman, 1989), information was taken from the transcripts and transferred onto a map or framework, allowing comparison by theme and case. The respondents' accounts were organised by categories and subcategories, suggested by the topic guides as well as new categories which emerged from analysis of transcripts.

Most qualitative papers don't contain detailed descriptions of the method employed but, as in this example, provide a reference to it. If interested enough the reader can consult the source themselves.

FIGURE 22.5   An example from the literature showing how authors summarise their general approach and refer the reader to a source for further details of the methodology, rather than give a detailed and comprehensive account of their methods.

Parents' perspectives on the MMR immunisation: a focus group study

Maggie Evans, Helen Stoddart, Louise Condon, Elaine Freeman, Marg Grizzel and Rebecca Mullen

Transcribed data were analysed using modified grounded theory techniques[15] by the research team. The transcripts were scrutinised, emerging themes and subthemes were agreed, and an initial coding index was developed. Sections of text were coded and these codes were applied to subsequent transcripts. Further codes were added as new themes emerged. Three members of the team coded some transcripts independently and a high level of consensus was achieved. Microsoft Word was used to develop individual files for each theme, allowing the text to be sorted and analysed in detail.

The reference '15' in this text supplies a detailed account of grounded theory for the interested reader.

FIGURE 22.6   Another, more comprehensive example from the literature, showing how authors summarise their general approach and refer the reader to a source for further details of the methodology.

23

Writing a Research Paper

If you are planning to present your findings as a research paper, then a good place to start looking for ideas is by browsing journals that you might want to target. Or even better, read our book, *Understanding Clinical Papers* (Bowers *et al.*, 2006).

Most research papers are built around a core structure – IMRAD, standing for Introduction, Methods, Results and Discussion. Let's look at what each of these in turn might entail.

THE INTRODUCTION

The trend in recent years, probably driven by the costs of publishing, has been for the introduction to be brief. Certainly it is not the place to undertake a review of the literature. For example, Figure 23.1 shows the sorts of points you might want to make in an introduction that will not generally be more than four paragraphs long. Some journals set out instructions about the length of the introduction, placing even more stringent restrictions on length.

IMRAD: the introduction

Importance   - clinical/public health
                                  - theoretical

What's been done before   - background/context

What's wrong with what's been done
                               - methodologically flawed
                               - incomplete
                               - doesn't generalize (age, setting, etc.)

End with questions or hypothesis

FIGURE 23.1   The main topics to be covered in a brief introduction to a clinical paper.

A Case Study: a few years ago we were involved in a research project that examined the association between life adversity and onset of breast cancer. The journal to which we submitted our manuscript expressed an interest in publishing the paper, but asked us to reduce its length and particularly the length of the introduction. What we did was write a list of the main points we wanted to make – shown in Figure 23.2.

Getting Started in Health Research, First Edition. David Bowers, Allan House and David Owens.
© 2011 David Bowers, Allan House and David Owens. Published 2011 by Blackwell Publishing Ltd.

---

stress and the onset of breast cancer

- it's a long-held belief that stress causes cancer, and lots of people still believe it

- the evidence is surprisingly weak

- recent studies in breast cancer have tried to answer the question by using a good measure and more robust research designs

- even so, the published studies are contradictory

- the latest study reported a strongly positive association, which attracted a lot of attention

- we wanted to replicate that study, because we thought it had methodological flaws (list)

FIGURE 23.2   Stress and the onset of breast cancer: the main points we wanted to cover in our introduction.

We then turned each point on the list into one or two grammatical sentences with references. This is what the introduction looked like (and you can spot our bullet points easily) when the paper was eventually published (see Figure 23.3).

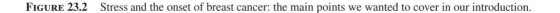

Stressful life events and difficulties and onset of breast cancer: case-control study

David Protheroe, Kim Turvey, Kieran Horgan, Eddie Benson, David Bowers, Allan House

Introduction

The belief that the onset of cancer may be associated with a stressful experience is found in the British, French and United States medical literature at least as far back as 1701. In a recent survey of South Australian women, 40% reported that they believed that stress was a cause of breast cancer. Research into the association, however, has methodological weaknesses.

Four recent studies of breast cancer have used the life events and difficulties schedule, a semi-structured interview of proved reliability: two examined the association between stress and relapse, and two examined the association between stress and onset of breast cancer. The results are not clear cut. In the most recent study, Chen *et al.* found that severe life events were associated with breast cancer, with an odds ratio of 11.6 after adjustment for confounders. The result provoked speculation about biological mechanisms for the effect, and widespread media coverage of the association between stress and cancer followed.

We have attempted to replicate the findings of Chen *et al.*, but with improvements in five areas of study design. Firstly, we included a larger sample of women presenting with a suspicious breast lump. Secondly, we obtained a consecutive series of women from a defined geographical area presenting with a breast lump, to reduce selection bias. Thirdly, we examined more social and physical risk factors for breast cancer to correct for potential confounding. Fourthly, we used two researchers who held regular consensus rating meetings to reduce observer bias. Finally, we examined the effect of the participant's knowledge of diagnosis on reporting of severe life events.

FIGURE 23.3   Stress and the onset of breast cancer: the introduction as it appeared in print with the main points covered in three paragraphs.

THE METHOD

How much detail you put in a methods section will depend very much on the journal for which you are writing. In general all journals want much the same structure, but how much they will want about each test or measure (for example) will depend upon whether it is a specialist or generalist journal, and whether it has separate facilities for on-line publication of technical details. Figure 23.4 shows some typical subheadings for a methods section of a research paper.

IMRAD: method

- study design
- setting
- sample
- measures
- statistical or qualitative software that was used
- statistical procedures used (the principles that were followed rather than the mere listing of tests)
- ethics and consent

FIGURE 23.4   Typical subheadings for the methods section of a research paper.

THE RESULTS

Because the main challenge in presenting your results is to get the best balance between text, tables, and figures, we will present our advice about the results section in Chapter 24.

THE DISCUSSION

Again, the current trend is for shorter discussions. If you want to demonstrate your erudition by summarising all the literature you have read, you will need to write a review article!

A typical discussion section therefore contains the components shown in Figures 23.5 and 23.6.

Once the main IMRAD structure is sorted out, you can start adding all the extras – most of which need to be written in the style of the journal in mind, adhering to any rules that they set out in their *Instructions to Authors* section – as for example in Figure 23.7.

AUTHORSHIP – WHICH AUTHORS WILL HAVE THEIR NAMES ON YOUR PAPER?

One topic we would particularly like to mention here is the decision about who is going to be an author on your paper. The key point is that every author on your paper must have made a substantial contribution at some stage in the research process. Some journals require that you describe the contribution of each author at the end of the paper, and what counts as 'substantial' might come as a surprise. For example, simply having obtained or provided funding for the research doesn't necessarily count, and neither does being head of the department in which the research was undertaken. We suggest that if you are being pressed to add names to the authors list for no good reason, so-called gift authorship, then you should consult a senior and independent advisor about how to resist.

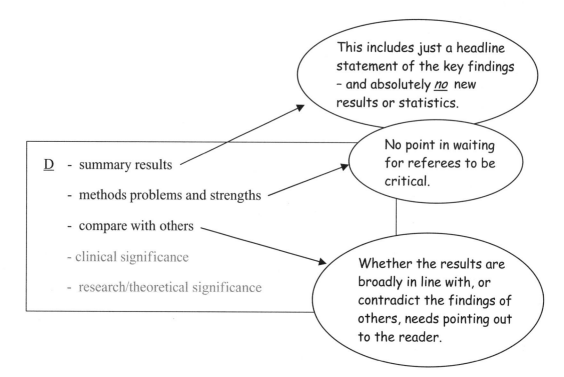

FIGURE 23.5   The main points to discover in your discussion.

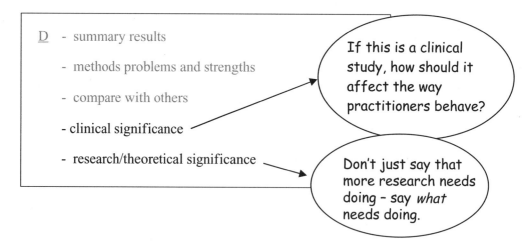

FIGURE 23.6   The main points to discover in your discussion – continued.

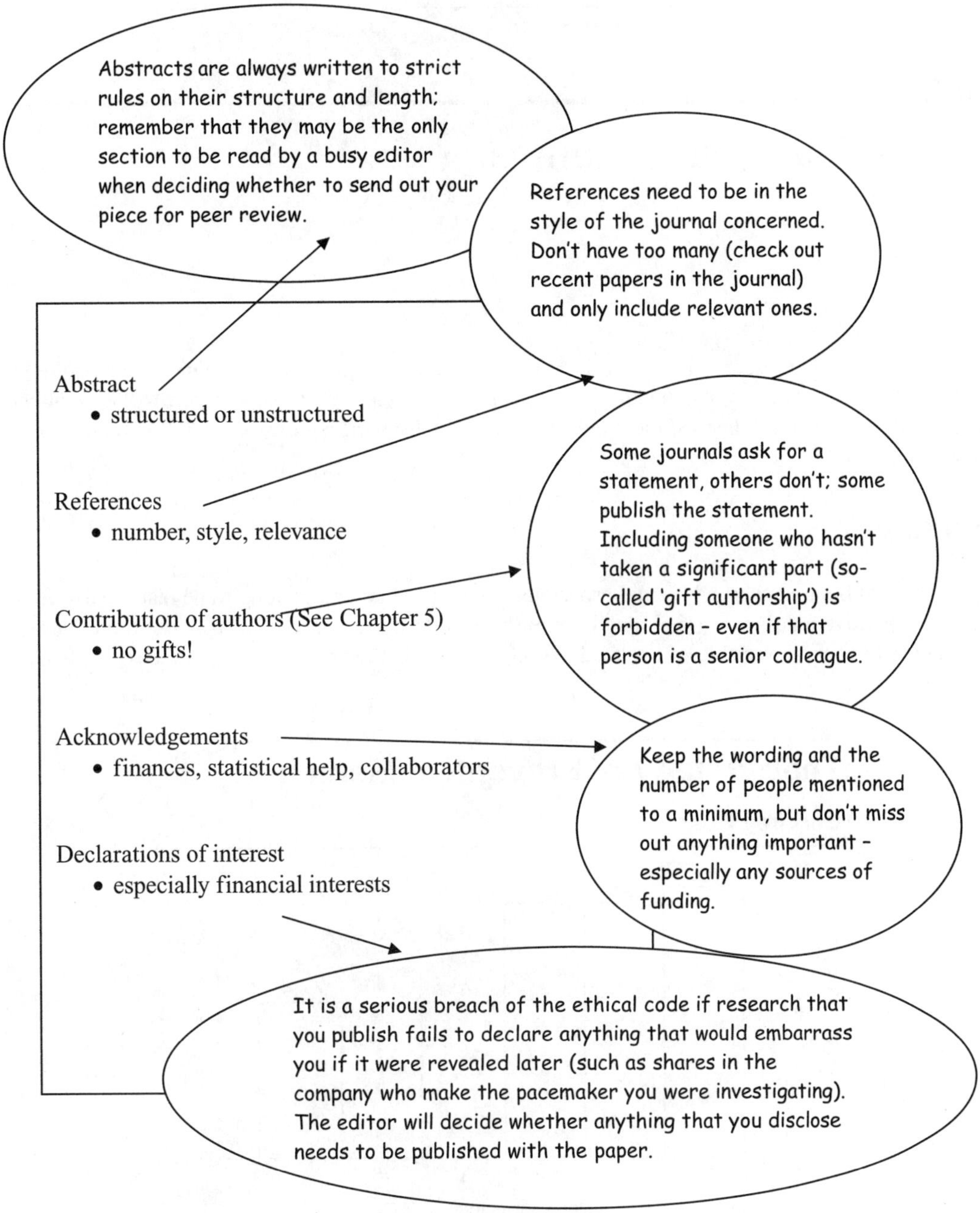

Abstracts are always written to strict rules on their structure and length; remember that they may be the only section to be read by a busy editor when deciding whether to send out your piece for peer review.

References need to be in the style of the journal concerned. Don't have too many (check out recent papers in the journal) and only include relevant ones.

Abstract
- structured or unstructured

References
- number, style, relevance

Some journals ask for a statement, others don't; some publish the statement. Including someone who hasn't taken a significant part (so-called 'gift authorship') is forbidden – even if that person is a senior colleague.

Contribution of authors (See Chapter 5)
- no gifts!

Acknowledgements
- finances, statistical help, collaborators

Keep the wording and the number of people mentioned to a minimum, but don't miss out anything important – especially any sources of funding.

Declarations of interest
- especially financial interests

It is a serious breach of the ethical code if research that you publish fails to declare anything that would embarrass you if it were revealed later (such as shares in the company who make the pacemaker you were investigating). The editor will decide whether anything that you disclose needs to be published with the paper.

FIGURE 23.7 Writing a paper – the extra bits (beyond IMRAD).

Be prepared to spend a lot of time preparing a paper for submission to a journal. You really must present it in the style of the journal that you have selected – and you must stick to their various rules. Doing so takes considerable attention to detail and more time than you expect. There is more about submission to journals in Chapter 27.

24

Setting Out Your Findings

Results are typically presented in one of three ways: text, tables and figures. A typical, even quite long, journal paper will contain only 4–6 tables and perhaps no figures, whilst a short report will have only one table. So be sparing! We will say something about each, but just to be contrary we will take them in reverse order.

FIGURES

Figures should be used sparingly – and especially if they need colour printing to be read easily, because they are expensive unless you are aiming to publish in an on-line resource. The best use for a figure is to show how two or more variables are related to each other, as in the example in Figure 24.1.

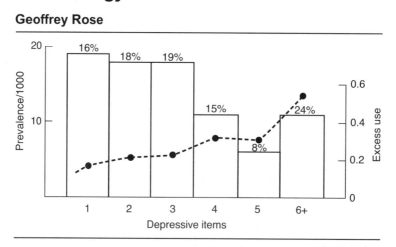

The Strategy of Preventive Medicine

Geoffrey Rose

FIGURE 24.1   An example of a figure showing the relations between three variables. Findings in a population survey of depression showing (1) the prevalence of reporting of various numbers of depressive features (bars), related to (2) the excess use of social supports above the rate for 'no depressive features' (broken line) and to (3) the proportions of this total excess attributable to different levels of depression (numbers above bars).

Getting Started in Health Research, First Edition. David Bowers, Allan House and David Owens.
© 2011 David Bowers, Allan House and David Owens. Published 2011 by Blackwell Publishing Ltd.

This apparently simple chart illustrates a key fact in epidemiology. First the graph shows that the relative risk of an outcome (use of social supports) goes up in direct relation to exposure to a risk (number of depressive symptoms). This association is shown by the dotted line. Second, it shows that the absolute risk of that outcome in a particular population doesn't necessarily go up in line with the relative risk – it depends upon the distribution of the risk. Here, for example, because not many people have very high numbers of depressive symptoms, more than half the social support in the sample was used by people with only mild or moderate depression.

Another use of figures is to show what happens to one or more variables over time – an especially important observation if two or more variables might be related as in Figure 24.2. This chart shows the association between new HIV diagnoses, HIV-1 viral load, and the number of individuals on HAART (highly active antiretroviral therapy) between 1996 and 2009, in British Columbia, Canada.

Association of highly active antiretroviral therapy coverage, population viral load, and yearly new HIV diagnoses in British Columbia, Canada: a population-based study

Julio S G Montaner, Vivian D Lima, Rolando Barrios, Benita Yip, Evan Wood, Thomas Kerr, Kate Shannon, P Richard Harrigan, Robert S Hogg

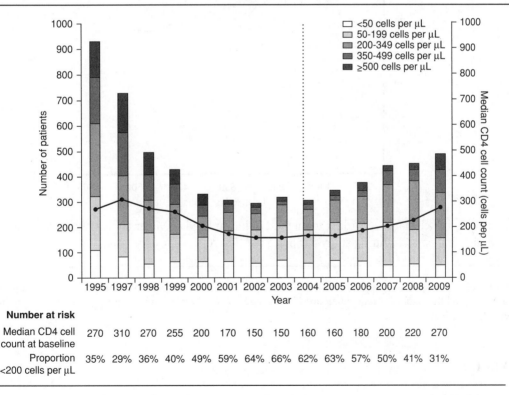

FIGURE 24.2   An example of a figure showing the relations between two variables across time and according to various policy changes.

Another common use of figures is to show the results of a survival analysis. There is no other way to show clearly the findings of such an analysis (Figure 24.3).

Hospital care and repetition following self-harm: a multicentre comparison of self-poisoning and self-injury

Lilley R, Owens D, Horrocks J, House A, Noble R, Bergen H, Hawton K, Casey D, Simkin S, Murphy E, Cooper J, Kapur N

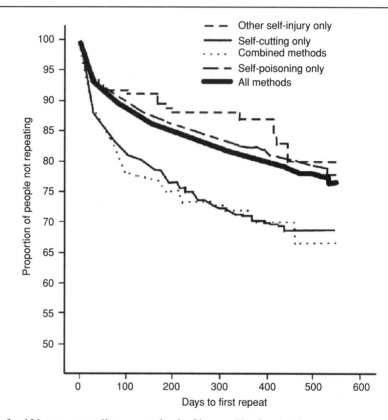

Repetition of self-harm according to method of harm: Kaplan-Meier curves represent time from the first episode during study period to the first repeat episode.

FIGURE 24.3   An example of a figure showing the findings from a survival analysis, with the overall survival pattern (thick line) and the values for four subgroups (from a study of self-harm examining time to repetition according to method of self-harm).

TABLES

Tables have a different use – they are an efficient way of showing large chunks of data when you don't want to display visually the relation between the variables. Figure 24.4 is a typical example from a general medical journal. One challenge in preparing tables is to decide how to present any statistical results in the table (Figure 24.5).

Antipsychotic drugs and risk of venous thromboembolism: nested case-control study

Chris Parker, medical statistician,[1] Carol Coupland, associate professor in medical statistics,[2] Julia Hippisley-Cox, professor of clinical epidemiology and general practice[2]

Table 3

  Characteristics of cases (patients with first ever record of venous thromboembolism) and matched controls at index date. Figures are numbers (percentages) unless stated otherwise

The two groups being compared.

Characteristics	Cases (n = 25 532)	Controls (n = 89 491)
Men	11 318 (44.3)	39 521 (44.2)
Women	14 214 (55.7)	49 970 (55.8)
Median (IQR) age (years)	67 (53-77)	67 (53-77)
Smoking status:		
Current smoker	4701 (18.4)	14 901 (16.7)
Not current smoker	17 531 (68.7)	59 130 (66.1)
Smoking status not recorded	3300 (12.9)	15 460 (17.3)
Body mass index (BMI):		
Not overweight (15.0-24.9)	6454 (25.3)	28 108 (31.4)
Overweight (25.0-29.9)	7390 (28.9)	24 869 (27.8)
Obese (30-50)	5629 (22.0)	12 527 (14.0)
No valid BMI recorded	6059 (23.7)	23 987 (26.8)
Fifth of socioeconomic status:		
1 (least deprived)	5798 (22.7)	21 898 (24.5)
2	5110 (20.0)	19 205 (21.5)
3	5233 (20.5)	18 592 (20.8)
4	5178 (20.3)	16 868 (18.8)
5 (most deprived)	4213 (16.5)	12 928 (14.4)
Median (IQR) months of previous data	164 (91-297)	167 (94-303)
Mental health conditions*:		
Schizophrenia	121 (0.5)	325 (0.4)
Bipolar disorder	73 (0.3)	198 (0.2)
Dementia	327 (1.3)	826 (0.9)
None of the above	25 011 (98.0)	88 142 (98.5)

FIGURE 24.4   An example of part of a large table showing lots of baseline data for the two groups being compared in a case-control study.

Hospital care and repetition following self-harm: a multicentre comparison of self-poisoning and self-injury

Lilley R, Owens D, Horrocks J, House A, Noble R, Bergen H, Hawton K, Casey D, Simkin S, Murphy E, Coop er J, Kapur N

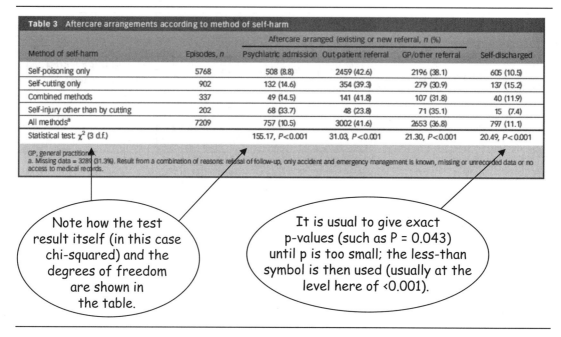

Table 3   Aftercare arrangements according to method of self-harm

Method of self-harm	Episodes, n	Aftercare arranged (existing or new referral, n (%))			
		Psychiatric admission	Out-patient referral	GP/other referral	Self-discharged
Self-poisoning only	5768	508 (8.8)	2459 (42.6)	2196 (38.1)	605 (10.5)
Self-cutting only	902	132 (14.6)	354 (39.3)	279 (30.9)	137 (15.2)
Combined methods	337	49 (14.5)	141 (41.8)	107 (31.8)	40 (11.9)
Self-injury other than by cutting	202	68 (33.7)	48 (23.8)	71 (35.1)	15 (7.4)
All methods[a]	7209	757 (10.5)	3002 (41.6)	2653 (36.8)	797 (11.1)
Statistical test: χ^2 (3 d.f.)		155.17, P<0.001	31.03, P<0.001	21.30, P<0.001	20.49, P<0.001

GP, general practitioner.
a. Missing data = 3289 (31.3%). Result from a combination of reasons: refusal of follow-up, only accident and emergency management is known, missing or unrecorded data or no access to medical records.

Note how the test result itself (in this case chi-squared) and the degrees of freedom are shown in the table.

It is usual to give exact p-values (such as P = 0.043) until p is too small; the less-than symbol is then used (usually at the level here of <0.001).

FIGURE 24.5   An example of a table showing the inclusion of statistical hypothesis testing (setting out the tests being used and the findings).

In this table four statistical tests were carried out and are reported. We chose to place the statistical test (the chi-squared test) at the bottom of each column because each test refers to the five rows of data immediately above it. We adhered to the journal's expectation (a good one) that the full test results should be set out: in this case the name of the test (X^2), the number of degrees of freedom (3 df in all of these four tests), the value for X^2 in each test, and the p-value. We would have given exact p-values (to 2 decimal places, P = 0.68 or P = 0.07 for example) but all p-values were so small in this example that they are simply reported as less than 0.001. The journal expects abbreviations to be explained in a footnote, and we have included within the footnote area some information about a large quantity of missing data.

In the next example from the same paper (Figure 24.6) the main findings are set out in terms of the odds ratio. The statistical information is, once again, set out in the table – as the 95% CI around each odds ratio. We prefer to say 0.35 (0.30 to 0.40), using the word 'to' instead of the dash, because the dash runs the risk of being misunderstood as a minus sign. But the journal has its own house style and altered the version that we sent in the manuscript.

Whether you are using tables or figures you should follow carefully the advice of the editor about where you place them in relation to the text. Do not embed them in the text of your manuscript just because that's what they are likely to look like when (if!) they are published. For most submissions, editors much prefer

Hospital care and repetition following self-harm: a multicentre comparison of self-poisoning and self-injury

Lilley R, Owens D, Horrocks J, House A, Noble R, Bergen H, Hawton K, Casey D, Simkin S, Murphy E, Cooper J, Kapur N

Table 2 Self-harm episodes and receipt of psychosocial assessment according to whether the method of harm was self-cutting only, adjusting for whether admitted to hospital or not

	Total, n	Psychosocial assessment			Odds ratio (95% CI)
		Proportion of sample assessed (%)	Assessed, n	Not assessed, n	
Total	5969	64.0	3822	2147	
Self-cutting only	832	42.1	350	482	0.35 (0.30–0.40)
All other methods	5137	67.6	3472	1665	
Admitted to hospital					
Self-cutting only	65	86.2	56	9	1.07 (0.53–2.18)
All other methods	2549	85.3	2175	374	
Not admitted to hospital					
Self-cutting only	767	38.3	294	473	0.62 (0.53–0.73)
All other methods	2588	50.1	1297	1291	
Mantel-Haenzel adjusted odds ratio					0.64 (0.54–0.75)

> Odds ratios are the main finding reported in this table, and each is shown with its confidence interval providing an estimate of its precision.

Figure 24.6   An example of a table showing the confidence intervals around the main findings.

figures and tables to be separate – each on its own page, and with its own legend clearly explaining what it is. One good test for yourself is to ask this question: if I dropped the page with this table (or figure) and its legend, separated from the text of my paper, would anybody who found it be able to work out what it shows? In other words, have I avoided lots of abbreviations, acronyms or initials to understand which the reader will need to keep looking in the text? Is the legend clear and self-explanatory?

Figure 24.7 is an illustration (fictitious but based on a real example) of how to get pretty much everything wrong. The table shows the odds ratios, along with their 95% CIs and p-values, for risk factors for stroke in males aged 60 and over. First the authors use a hyphen in the confidence intervals and not the word 'to', which would have been better practice. Second they write 'NS' for 'Not Significant' for the p-values (last column) – it would be much more helpful to give the exact value. Finally they don't explain the meaning of TMS or NSAIDs anywhere (for instance in a footnote to the table).

One last word about tables. As in the example below, when you produce a table in a word-processing package what you usually get is a grid that helps you enter numbers. For a really simple example like the one above that may do, but for more complicated tables with several rows or columns you should use dividing lines more sparingly and make better use of white space to make the data easily readable. The examples in Figures 24.5 and 24.6 show how the journals tend to use only a few horizontal lines.

Odds ratios for stroke in men aged 60+ related to recent activities

Event	OR (95% CI)	P
Running	2.4 (0.5–10)	NS
Playing contact sport	3.5 (0.6–11)	NS
Playing squash	15 (4.8 to 289)	< 0.001
Excessive steroid use	2.9 (0.5–12)	NS
TMS	20 (2.9–217)	< 0.005
Excessive use of NDSAIDs	4.5 (0.9–21)	NS

FIGURE 24.7   An example of a table that has deficiencies in its construction.

TEXT

Once you have your tables and figures sorted out, the job of the text becomes clearer. First it can be used to draw the reader's attention to key points in the tables, and adding some additional information, as in the following example (see Figure 24.8).

Molecular Markers and Death From Prostate Cancer

Concato J, Jain D, Uchio E, Risch H, Li WW, Wells CK

RESULTS
Baseline Factors

Table 1 shows the characteristics of 1172 men with a prostate cancer diagnosis from 1991 to 1995. The median age at diagnosis was 72 years; 127 men (11%) were black, 672 (57%) had no or mild comorbid conditions, 1040 (89%) had clinically localized cancer, and 711 (61%) had moderately differentiated tumors (Gleason score, 5 to 7); and the median PSA level was 10.0 µg/L. Initial treatment included prostatectomy or radiation therapy in 632 (54%) men, hormonal ablation in 215 (18%) men, and watchful waiting or no treatment in 325 (28%) men. Among the latter group, 106 (33%) subsequently received therapy. The w statistics for concordance (21) were 0.77 for comorbid conditions, 0.92 for histologic grade, and 0.80 for immunohistochemical readings.

Table 1 also shows results of the immunohistochemical analyses.

FIGURE 24.8   An extensive legend to a table can point out its main features.

A second use of text is to present data that aren't there at all in the tables, and to describe the approach to statistical analysis and present details of results.

If your paper describes a qualitative research project, then it is likely that your results will be presented largely or entirely as text. You will probably have noticed that in this situation many authors include verbatim quotes from the participants – taken, for example, from transcripts of interviews. This can be a useful approach but only if these quotations add something; all too often we notice that badly chosen quotations simply repeat a point made in the text.

In Figure 24.9 we reproduce a quotation from a health professional interviewed about his or her approach to counselling women who have a positive antenatal test for a particular genetic disorder (sickle cell disease). The quotation sheds light on the consultant's thinking in a way that a textual summary by the author would not do and allows us to see something of how the process might actually unfold in the clinic.

Screening and Counselling for Sickle Cell Disorders and Thalassaemia: The Experience of Parents and Health Professionals

KARL ATKIN, WAQAR I.U. AHMAD and ELIZABETH N. ANIONWU

I suppose I do not outline all the options as being neutral, because I think maybe the families don't understand how bad it is going to be to have thalassaemia. I do go out of the way to make the option of antenatal diagnosis and try to stop them, you know. 'Keep our fingers crossed', is the likely response and I like to encourage them to think more seriously about the other options. But I do not believe that there is any such thing as value free counselling, it is not about a neutral choice and I feel I need to lean on their background prejudices by encouraging them towards . . . one view rather than another. So I have to admit that I do advocate termination, I suppose.

FIGURE 24.9   A quotation from a health professional interviewed about his or her approach to counselling women who have a positive antenatal test for a particular genetic disorder (sickle cell disease).

What you may want to put in text is so diverse that, if you aren't an experienced writer, we would strongly advise you of two things: first, get an experienced author to give you some help, and second, look in your target journal, reading now not for the content of any paper you glance at but to check *how* rather than *what* the authors have presented.

25

Writing Your Discussion

Although the Discussion section of a paper very rarely has subheadings, it is nonetheless true that it usually follows a fairly conventional format.

First comes a summary statement of your key findings. The trick here is to avoid two common errors – simply repeating a chunk of your results section, or slipping in new results (or statistics) as an afterthought. The best way to approach this summary is to write it like a press release or news summary – what is the take-home message for your readers? Figure 25.1 is an example of a particularly informal presentation of a paper's key findings.

Dynamic spread of happiness in a large social network: longitudinal analysis of the Framington Heart Study social network

James H. Fowler, Nicholas Christakis

Discussion

While there are many determinants of happiness, whether an individual is happy also depends on whether others in the individual's social network are happy. Happy people tend to be located in the centre of their local social networks and in large clusters of other happy people. The happiness of an individual is associated with the happiness of people up to three degrees removed in the social network. Happiness in other words, is not merely a function of individual experience or individual choice but is also a property of groups of people. Indeed, changes in individual happiness can ripple through social networks and generate large-scale structure in the network, giving rise to clusters of happy and unhappy individuals. These results are even more remarkable considering . . .

FIGURE 25.1   The start of a discussion often summarises the main findings.

Second, it is usually a good idea to review the strengths and weaknesses of your study. It is tempting to concentrate on the strengths, and certainly it is worth pointing out the steps you have taken to produce research that is methodologically stronger that its predecessors. But it is worth also highlighting the

---

Getting Started in Health Research, First Edition. David Bowers, Allan House and David Owens.
© 2011 David Bowers, Allan House and David Owens. Published 2011 by Blackwell Publishing Ltd.

weaknesses and limitations of what you have done. If you don't, the editor's reviewers will (!) And if you do outline your own weaknesses, you can use your discussion of strengths to point out why the problems do not matter too much. Some journals put parts of the discussion in a separate text box, as shown in Figure 25.2.

Exploring the impact of patient views on 'appropriate' use of services and help seeking: a mixed method study

Joy Adamson, Yoav Ben-Shlomo, Nish Chaturvedi and Jenny Donovan

How this fits in

There are commonly held views relating to what constitutes appropriate and inappropriate use of finite NHS resources. Little is known about how and why such views have an impact on consultation patterns. The study indicated that strong views relating to unnecessary service use were not predictive of reported help-seeking. Responders tend to consider other people as time-wasters, but not themselves. Perceptions that individuals use health services inappropriately are unlikely to explain differences in consultation behaviours. While patients may consult for seemingly trivial conditions, they rationalise why their behaviour is not unnecessary.

FIGURE 25.2   Text boxes are often used for punchy or 'take-home' messages.

In a more conventional discussion in the text the authors will outline the strengths and novelties of their study, to indicate its value (see for example Figure 25.3).

Aspirin Use and Survival After Diagnosis of Colorectal Cancer

Andrew T. Chan, Shugi Ogino, Charles S. Fuchs

Our study has several important strengths. First, we used prospectively collected data on aspirin use. Thus, we were able to minimize potential bias related to differential recall of aspirin use according to disease activity, and any errors in recall would have tended to attenuate rather than exaggerate true associations. Second, we obtained data on aspirin use both before and after cancer diagnosis. This permitted us to disentangle the effect of aspirin use after diagnosis from aspirin use before diagnosis. We considered the possibility that regular aspirin users who develop colorectal cancer simply acquire tumors that are biologically less aggressive. However, the benefit of regular aspirin use was largely restricted to patients who initiated aspirin use following cancer diagnosis; after adjusting for postdiagnosis aspirin use, regular aspirin use before cancer diagnosis was not associated with any reduction in colorectal cancer or overall mortality. Finally, since all participants were health professionals, the accuracy of self-reported aspirin use is likely to be high and more likely to reflect actual consumption of these largely over-the-counter medications.

FIGURE 25.3   A typical discussion includes an account of the main strengths of a study.

Less common but just as important is a discussion of the weaknesses of a study; here is such a consideration from the same authors who have just outlined the strengths of their study (see Figure 25.4)

Aspirin Use and Survival After Diagnosis of Colorectal Cancer

Andrew T. Chan, Shugi Ogino, Charles S. Fuchs

Several limitations of this study warrant comment. First, our study was observational and aspirin use was self-selected. Thus, despite the strong biological plausibility of our results, it is possible that our findings could be related to the reason for which participants used aspirin. However, most participants reported using aspirin primarily for analgesia.[27] During much of the study period, data regarding an association between aspirin and colorectal neoplasia were also not widely available, suggesting that it is unlikely participants took aspirin for the purpose of cancer prevention. Moreover, an analysis adjusting for an individual's propensity to use aspirin also did not materially change our results. We also cannot completely exclude the possibility that aspirin use may be reflective of other occult predictors for improved prognosis. However, we did not observe any significant association between aspirin use and other predictors of cancer outcome and our findings remained unchanged after adjusting for other potential risk factors for colorectal cancer mortality. Finally, the differential effect of aspirin according to COX-2 expression is consistent with a causal mechanism. To minimize any bias by occult recurrence, we also performed a secondary analysis in which we excluded deaths within 12 months of the aspirin assessment and continued to observe a significant influence of regular aspirin use on patient outcome.

FIGURE 25.4   The discussion of high-quality papers also includes an account of the main weaknesses of a study.

Third, the discussion needs to place your results (taking account of their strengths and weaknesses) in context. How do they sit with the rest of the literature on this topic? There are three broad ways you can place your findings:

- There is a broad consensus in the literature, to which your own findings contribute – they are confirmatory.
- There is a consensus in the literature that your results contradict, or they shed new light on a problem or add new knowledge – they are ground breaking.
- There is no consensus and your results support one position more than another, or are themselves contradictory – the meaning of your results is debatable.

Finally and most challenging is the need to say something about *implications for practice*. On the one hand, if your results are important they should lead to some change. But realistically, very little research is so important that on its own it leads to change in practice. One way to tackle this dilemma is to consider not the idea of change in practice but the balance of probabilities (or confidence one might have) that one course of action rather than another is correct. An example of an implications discussion is given in Figure 25.5.

Cardiovascular disease

Folic acid, homocysteine, and cardiovascular disease: judging causality in the face of inconclusive trial evidence

Denis S. Wald, Joan K. Morris, Malcolm Law, Nicholas J. Wald

The table shows the summary results from the meta-analyses of the cohort studies, the genetic polymorphism studies, and the randomised trials, the first two adjusted to the average homocysteine decrease of 3.3 _mol/l for ischaemic heart disease and 2.9 _mol/l for stroke, observed in the randomised trials. The cohort and genetic studies give similar results even though they do not share the same sources of error. The dose-response relation in the genetic studies is particularly relevant in suggesting a causal effect. The summary estimate from the trials is consistent with a short term protective effect of 12% on ischaemic heart disease events and 22% on stroke, or a larger long term effect. The conclusion that homocysteine is a cause of cardiovascular disease explains the observations from all the different types of study, even if the results from one type of study are, on their own, insufficient to reach that conclusion. No single alternative explanation can account for all the observations. Since folic acid reduces homocysteine concentrations, to an extent dependent on background folate levels, it follows that increasing folic acid consumption will reduce the risk of heart attack and stroke by an amount related to the homocysteine reduction achieved. We therefore take the view that the evidence is now sufficient to justify action on lowering homocysteine concentrations, although the position should be reviewed as evidence from ongoing clinical trials emerges.

FIGURE 25.5   Although most papers do not illustrate their discussion with a table, they will put their results in context.

When you have finished writing up your research, you will probably want to either submit it as a research thesis for a postgraduate degree, or get it published in a journal. In the next two chapters we will consider the ramifications of each of these in turn.

26

Writing a Thesis or Other Report

For many people, the first piece of scientific writing they do is not a research paper but a thesis, a dissertation (a small thesis, usually the last part of a taught degree), or a research report for their department or for a funding body. This can be a substantial advantage because such a thesis should, according to the requirements of the degree being studied, be closely supervised. What are the differences in approach? We'll discuss the thesis/dissertation first, and deal with the research report after this.

A THESIS OR DISSERTATION

The IMRAD approach serves as a useful basis but it will need modification:

The *introduction* will be more extensive, exploring theory and reviewing in more detail what has gone before. With the advent of systematic reviewing, you will need to decide whether you can justify a non-systematic account of the literature. The alternative is to write a very brief scene-setting introduction and then make your first study a systematic literature review. Even if the review of the literature is not a full systematic review, you might consider including your search strategies as an appendix to the thesis.

The *questions* you asked will require more justification than in a paper, and they will be framed as aims and hypotheses in a more formal way. The *methods* section will have to be greatly expanded. One of the substantial differences between a paper and a thesis is that in the latter the methods used have to be justified as well as described. Thus it is worth starting with a section on methodological considerations before going on to present what you actually did in detail – the measures you used and the process and timetable of assessments. We find, in first drafts of theses on which we are asked to comment, that the writer has been much too spare with the description of methods. The primary purpose of a thesis is a demonstration of the student's learning (and even an experienced clinician is a 'student' when undertaking a doctoral or master's degree); describing exactly what was done is one of the best ways of providing evidence of the learning that has occurred. We should add here that, again in our experience, the method is the only section where research students tend to be too brief: in all other sections the tendency is to ramble on with insufficient structure and discipline.

The *results* section in a thesis or dissertation will usually allow for the setting out of substantially more of the findings than would be permissible in a journal paper. This is likely to mean more tables and figures than in a paper; each will need careful construction – after deliberation about whether it adds substantially to the story being woven by the author. A common mistake is to spray a huge quantity of numerical findings or qualitative quotes on to the pages. In so doing the story is lost and the reader

Getting Started in Health Research, First Edition. David Bowers, Allan House and David Owens.
© 2011 David Bowers, Allan House and David Owens. Published 2011 by Blackwell Publishing Ltd.

will become bored and will lose the thread of the story (and perhaps the will to live). A variation on this error is to display numerical findings in tables and then repeat them in figures – as barcharts, perhaps. Instead, figures are best reserved for the display of findings where tables cannot achieve the same level of explanation (see Chapter 24).

The *discussion* section follows the same basic format as for a paper (Chapter 25) although it will be more detailed, especially in setting out the strengths and weaknesses of the study's design and conduct. Examiners of a dissertation or thesis will want to see that the candidate for the degree has understood his or her limitations – although you should not be timid about asserting any strengths, especially when drawing comparison with other people's published work.

Dinesh, for example, will find that some of the data that he wishes to collect are not available – because staff in the busy emergency department haven't recorded all of the relevant facts. He needs to acknowledge this failing in his discussion. But he should be prepared to point out a strength of his work too: that most of the earlier research on his topic (hospital attendance as a result of self-harm) has been based on patients who have stayed long enough to be admitted to the inpatient unit. Inpatient care means that the recording of data is much more comprehensive than is the case for those seen only in the emergency department, but studies of inpatients deal only with a restricted study population that excludes the many patients who go home directly from the emergency department.

The discussion section of a thesis might also be the place for some consideration of theoretical implications of the study's findings. Journal papers will usually not be the place for this kind of speculation but it may be an important part of a thesis; this is a particular matter for the supervisor's advice.

Some theses bring together several inter-related projects – in a way that a journal paper would never do. In this case, the overall structure of your thesis will require some thought. Probably the best structure in those circumstances is to conceive each chapter as a self-contained report and then write linking sections, with an over-arching introduction and an over-arching discussion setting the context at the start and end.

Because the details of thesis content and formatting vary so much, we suggest strongly that you:

- Consult your university's requirements and if they provide one (as most do) use a word-processing template;
- Visit your library and examine past successful theses; they will usually allow you to peruse examples while you are visiting the library;
- Get advice from an experienced and critical writer – who may or may not be your academic supervisor.

Leave enough time! Hofstadter's law applies here.[1] We have elected to say no more here about theses because the local arrangements vary greatly. Our very strong advice is that you rely on repeated consultation of your local requirements for the thesis together with regular supervision. There are a number of books devoted to the writing of the thesis; you might find one or more of them useful. Since none of us used one ourselves during the completion (many years ago) of our theses, we do not wish to make a specific recommendation.

WRITING A RESEARCH REPORT

The introduction to such reports often contains more policy or other context to the research.

The language will typically need to be modified for an audience that may not be from your speciality area, and indeed may not be from a scientific background. You must learn to write simple clear

---

[1] Hofstadter's Law: 'It always takes longer than you expect, even when you take Hofstadter's Law into account.'

English – many funders of research now require a lay summary in their reports and on their application forms for funding (see Chapter 15).

When writing research reports you will find that figures and tables may be embedded in the body of the text and the use of mini summaries or text boxes can be a good idea.

27

Dealing With Journals

The first decision you have to make once your paper is near completion is: to which journal will I submit it for publication? Most of us want to be widely read so we aspire to publish in the most popular journals. One measure of popularity is the so-called *impact factor*, which reflects how often papers published in the journal are cited (on average) by other people. There are, however, disadvantages in trying to publish in high impact factor journals:

- Their popularity means that there is a lot of competition from other researchers, so your chances of acceptance are lower;
- Popularity also means pressure on space so these journals tend to publish large numbers of relatively short papers per issue;
- In many areas wide readership is achieved by appealing to a diverse population of subscribers, so your paper may be seen as too specialist.

Your best bet is to browse likely journals looking for ones that publish similar articles to the one you are writing. Your own references will draw on these likely journals. You should also get advice from a senior colleague with publishing experience about which journals to aim for first.

Once you have selected a target journal, you will need to tailor your manuscript to fit that journal's *Instructions to Authors*.

These instructions are pretty much all available on-line now, and will not only tell you how the journal wants manuscripts presented but will also guide you through the submission process.

A really helpful website is http://mulford.utoledo.edu/instr/ which provides links to all the instructions to authors' pages of common journals (see Figure 27.1).

Once you have got a draft manuscript together, while you are preparing it along the lines of your chosen target journal, there are a number of additional tasks:

(1) Get constructive criticism **on at least two drafts** from colleagues.
(2) Edit for length (word count) and numbers of tables, figures and references allowed by your target journal.
(3) Check carefully – for spelling errors and typos.
(4) Check formatting – page numbering, typeface and so on. Do not use right justification in your manuscript – it may look superficially neat but it actually makes reading harder! If you look at the right margin of a typical book you will see that the printer has inserted breaks in the last word of many lines – in order to achieve a pleasing and even spacing of words; you will not have the skill to do that so left justification is the safer and preferred option.

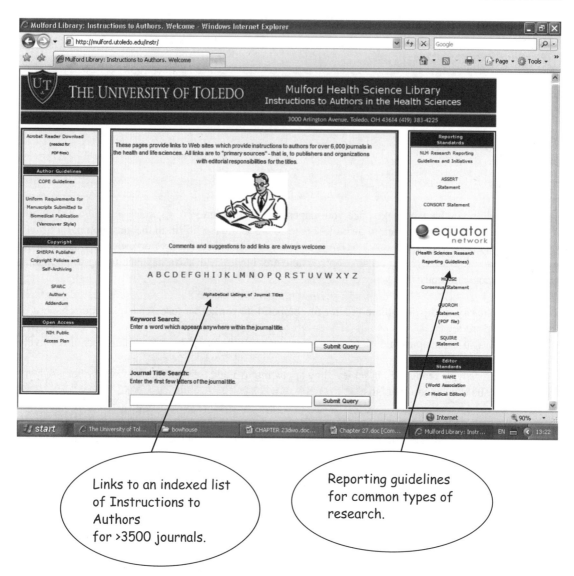

FIGURE 27.1   A useful on-line resource that links to authors for all major health-related journals.

Whether you submit electronically or by sending paper copies, you will need to write a covering letter. There are really only two things you need to say in this letter – why the editor should publish your paper, and that it has not been published elsewhere and is not about to be.

The covering letter Anna wrote is shown in Figure 27.2.

Occasionally you will get a very quick reply saying the journal is so certain they will not publish that they do not intend to ask for referees comments. Shrug your shoulders and try elsewhere – there is no point in arguing.

More typically, you will wait a few weeks and then get a letter from the journal. Sometimes again it contains an outright rejection. The reasons will be outlined and often accompanied by more detailed

The Editor
British Journal of General Practice

Dear Sir,

Thank you for considering this paper. We believe it will be of interest to your readers because it is topical and deals with a clinically important subject, and because we make a number of practical suggestions that will be of use to clinicians working in primary care.

The paper has not been published, and is not under consideration for publication, in any other journal.

Yours faithfully,

FIGURE 27.2   Letters to editors should be brief and to the point, while explaining why the paper is worth looking at.

feedback from referees. Do not despair! You can use the referees' comments to help you improve your manuscript and resubmit elsewhere. Do not do so immediately, instead:

– Take a couple of weeks to reflect
– Discuss with your co-authors
– Revise and make sure you are confident you have dealt with all the criticisms
– Choose a different journal with a lower rejection rate.

If you are lucky you will get a letter that says something rather different. Figure 27.3 is the letter Anna received.

Dear Dr . . . ,

Thank you for allowing us to review your manuscript. I am afraid that I cannot accept it in its current form but if you are prepared to make changes then I would be willing to consider it again.

In particular you will see that my reviewers thought there were too many quotations from the patients you interviewed, which made your paper rather long and repetitive. The advice to clinicians needs to be presented more succinctly – perhaps as a series of bullet points or in a text box.

I attach my reviewers other comments. If you decide to resubmit then please provide a covering letter outlining the changes you have made in the light of these comments.

Yours sincerely,

FIGURE 27.3   Many first time authors are put off by a letter like this. In reality it is an invitation to rewrite and try again.

This is not an agreement to publish but it is the next-best-thing. What it means is that if Anna makes the changes suggested, then the editor will be well disposed towards the paper. Under similar circumstances you should make all the changes suggested by referees, except where two referees say diametrically opposite things. If they do you will need to seek the editor's advice. If you think a referee has made a mistake or misunderstood a point say so politely in your response to the editor. Be careful if you choose to argue with referees, it never goes down well and it is highly likely that the real problem is that you did not explain clearly what you had done or found.

Otherwise – nothing to do except sit back and wait for the proofs to arrive! Oh, and start planning your next piece of research . . .

Further Reading

Adamson J, Ben-Shlomo Y, Chaturvedi N, Donovan J (2009) Exploring the impact of patient views on 'appropriate' use of services and help seeking: a mixed method study. *British Journal of General Practice;* 59.

Altman D G, Bland J M (1999) How to randomise. *British Medical Journal;* 319.

Atkin K, Ahmad W I U, Anionwu E N (1998) Screening and counselling for sickle cell disorders and thalassaemia: the experience of parents and health professionals. *Social Science & Medicine;* 47.

Bolliger C T, Zellweger J-P, Danielsson T *et al.* (2000) Smoking reduction with oral nicotine inhalers: double blind, randomised clinical trial of efficacy and safety. *British Medical Journal;* 321.

Bonita R, Beaglehole R, Kjellstrom T (2006) *Basic Epidemiology* (2nd edn), World Health Organization, Geneva. Chapter 3.

Bourhis J, Overgaard J, Audry H *et al.*, on behalf of the Meta-Analysis of Radiotherapy in Carcinomas of Head and neck (MARCH) Collaborative Group (2006) Hyperfractionated or accelerated radiotherapy in head and neck cancer: a meta-analysis. *The Lancet;* 368.

Bowers D (2008) *Medical Statistics from Scratch* (2nd edn), John Wiley & Sons, Ltd, Chichester.

Bowers D, House A O, Owens D W (2006) *Understanding Clinical Papers* (2nd edn), John Wiley & Sons, Ltd, Chichester.

Burkey Y, Black M, Reeve H (1997). Patients' views on their discharge from follow-up in outpatient clinics: qualitative study. *British Medical Journal;* 315.

Campbell R, Pound P, Pope C *et al.* (2003) Evaluating meta-ethnography: a synthesis of qualitative research on lay experiences of diabetes and diabetes care. *Social Science & Medicine;* 56.

Chan A T, Ogino S, Fuchs C S (2009) Aspirin use and survival after diagnosis of colorectal cancer. *Journal of the American Medical Association;* 302.

Chapman K R, Kesten S, Szalai J P (1994) Regular vs as-needed inhaled salbutamol in asthma control. *The Lancet;* 343.

Collerton J, Davies K, Jagger C *et al.* (2009) Health and disease in 85 year olds: baseline findings from the Newcastle 85+ cohort study. *British Medical Journal;* 339.

Concato J, Jain D, Uchio E *et al.* (2009) Molecular markers and death from prostate cancer. *Annals of Internal Medicine;* 150.

Duke T, Poka H, Dale F *et al.* (2002) Chloramphenicol versus benzylpenicillin and gentamicin for the treatment of severe pneumonia in children in Papua New Guinea: a randomised trial. *The Lancet;* 359.

Choi H K, Hernán M A, Seeger J D, Robins J M, Wolfe F (2002) Methotrexate and mortality in patients with rheumatoid arthritis: a prospective study. *The Lancet;* 359.

Ellenberg J H, Nelson K B (1980) Sample selection and the natural history of disease. Studies of febrile seizures. *Journal of the American Medical Association;* 243, April 4 [adapted].

Evans A T, Husain S, Durairaj L, Sadowski L S, Charles-Damte M, Wang Y (2002) Azithromycin for acute bronchitis: a randomised, double-blind, controlled trial. *The Lancet;* 359.

Evans M, Stoddart H, Condon L *et al.* (2001) Parents' perspectives on the MMR immunisation: a focus group study. *British Journal of General Practice;* 51.

Fowler J H, Christakis N A (2008) Dynamic spread of happiness in a large social network: longitudinal analysis of the Framingham Heart Study. *British Medical Journal;* 337.

Gordis L (2008) *Epidemiology* (4th edn), W B Saunders, Philadelphia. Chapters 7–10.

Getting Started in Health Research, First Edition. David Bowers, Allan House and David Owens.
© 2011 David Bowers, Allan House and David Owens. Published 2011 by Blackwell Publishing Ltd.

Hamilton M, Corwin P, Gower S, Rogers S (2004) Why do parents choose not to immunise their children? *The New Zealand Medical Journal*; 117.

Hennekens C H, Buring J E (1987) *Epidemiology in Medicine*, Little, Brown & Co., Boston. Chapters 2, 5–8.

Hippisley-Cox J, Pringle M, Hammersley V *et al.* (2001) Antidepressants as a risk factor for ischaemic heart disease: case-control study in primary care. *British Medical Journal*; 323.

Kühne T, Imbach P, Bolton-Maggs P H B *et al.*, for the Intercontinental Childhood ITP Study Group (2001) Newly diagnosed idiopathic thrombocytopenic purpura in childhood: an observational study. *The Lancet*; 358.

Langan S M, Smeeth L, Hubbard R *et al.* (2008) Bullous pemphigoid and pemphigus vulgaris – incidence and mortality in the UK: population based cohort. *British Medical Journal*; 337.

Lilley R, Owens D, Horrocks J *et al.* (2008) Hospital care and repetition following self-harm: multicentre comparison of self-poisoning and self-injury. *The British Journal of Psychiatry*; 192.

Ludermir A B, Lewis G, Valongueiro S A, Barreto de Arauja T V, Araya R (2010) Violence against women by their intimate partner during pregnancy and postnatal depression: a prospective cohort study. *The Lancet*; 376.

Meaney P A, Nadkarni V M, Cook E F *et al.*, for the American Heart Association National Registry of Cardiopulmonary Resuscitation Investigators (2006) Higher survival rates among younger patients after pediatric intensive care unit cardiac arrests. *Pediatrics*; 118.

Montaner J S G, Lima V D, Barrios R *et al.* (2010) Association of highly active antiretroviral therapy coverage, population viral load, and yearly new HIV diagnoses in British Columbia, Canada: a population-based study. *The Lancet;* 376.

Naumburg E, Bellocco R, Cnattingius S, Hall P, Ekbom A (2000) Prenatal ultrasound examinations and risk of childhood leukaemia: a case-control study. *British Medical Journal*; 320.

Nichter M, Nichter M, Adrian S *et al.* (2008) Smoking and harm-reduction efforts among postpartum women. *Qualitative Health Research*; 18.

Parker C, Coupland C, Hippisley-Cox J (2010) Antipsychotic drugs and risk of venous thromboembolism: nested case-control study. *British Medical Journal*; 341.

Pope C, Mays N (Eds) (2006) *Qualitative Research in Health Care* (3rd edn), Blackwell Publishing, Oxford. Chapters 1–4.

Protheroe D, Turvey K, Horgan K *et al.* (1999) Stressful life events and difficulties and onset of breast cancer: case-control study. *British Medical Journal*; 319.

Riegelman R K (2005) *Studying a Study and Testing a Test* (5th edn), Lippincott, Williams & Wilkins, Philadelphia. Section I: Chapters 2–12.

Ritchie J, Lewis J (Eds) (2003) *Qualitative Research Practice*, Sage, London. Chapters 3 and 4.

Roberts D, Dalziel S (2006) Antenatal corticosteroids for accelerating fetal lung maturation for women at risk of preterm birth. *Cochrane Database of Systematic Reviews*; 3.

Romero-Corral A, Montori V M, Somers V K *et al.* (2006) Association of bodyweight with total mortality and with cardiovascular events in coronary artery disease: a systematic review of cohort studies. *The Lancet*; 368.

Rose G (1993) *The Strategy of Preventative Medicine*, Oxford University Press, Oxford.

Rossignol J-F, Abu-Zekry M, Hussein A, Santoro M G (2006) Effect of nitazoxanide for the treatment of severe rotavirus diarrhoea: a randomised double-blind placebo-controlled trial. *The Lancet*; 368.

Rydström I, Dalheim-Englund A-C, Holritz-Rasmussen B, Möller C, Sandman P-O (2005) Asthma – quality of life for Swedish children. *Journal of Clinical Nursing*; 14.

Saravanan P, Davidson N, Schmidt E B, Calder P C (2010) Cardiovascular effects of marine omega-3 fatty acids. *The Lancet*; 376.

Sari A B-A, Sheldon T A, Cracknell A, Turnbull A (2007) Sensitivity of routine system for reporting patient safety incidents in an NHS hospital: retrospective patient case note review. *British Medical Journal*; 334:79.

Sackett D (2000) Experts: off with their heads. *British Medical Journal*; 320.

Schrader H, Stovner L J, Helde G, Sand T, Bovim G (2001) Prophylactic treatment of migraine with angiotensin converting enzyme inhibitor (lisinopril): randomised, placebo controlled, crossover study. *British Medical Journal*; 322.

Silverman D. (2005) *Doing Qualitative Research* (2nd edn), Sage, London. Chapters 4, 8, 9.

Streiner D L, Norman G R (1998) *PDQ Epidemiology* (2nd edn), B C Decker Inc., Hamilton. Chapter 3.

Sword W, Busser D, Ganann R, McMillan T, Swinton M (2008) Women's care-seeking experiences after referral for postpartum depression. *Qualitative Health Research*; 18.

Thomson A B, Campbell A J, Irvine D S *et al.* (2001) Semen quality and spermatozoal DNA integrity in survivors of childhood cancer: a case-control study. *The Lancet*; 360.

Wald D S, Wald N J, Morris J K, Law M, Wald N J (2006). Folic acid, homocysteine, and cardiovascular disease: judging causality in the face of inconclusive trial evidence. *British Medical Journal*; 333.

Wannamethee S G, Lever A F, Shaper A G, Whincup P H (1997) Serum potassium, cigarette smoking, and mortality in middle-aged men. *The American Journal of Epidemiology*; 145.

Index

Page numbers in *italics* denote figures.

aims of research 3
analysis
    qualitative research 144–7, *144–7*
    quantitative research 136–43, *137–41*
        baseline tables 136, *137*
        choice of method 85–6

Bland-Altman test 86

case-control studies 43
    control subjects 51, 53, *53*
case-mix measures 63
chain sampling 57–8
charities, funding by 98
chi-squared test 86
choice of method 45–6
clinical audit *101*
clinical collaborator 36–7
clinical databases 50, *51*
clinical trials 43
cluster sampling 48–9, *49*
  multistage 49
Cochrane Library 26
cohort studies 43
computers
    quantitative data 127–8, *128*
    security of 123
    use in data collection 122–3
confidence intervals 77, 86
confounding 68–75, 141–3, *142, 143*
    dealing with 70–5
      matching 72, *72*
      randomisation 74–5, *74*
      restriction 70–1, *71*
      statistical adjustment 73–4, *73*
    definition of 68–9, *69*
    example of 69–70, *70*
consecutive sampling 50, *50*
consent form 105–9

contingency table analysis 86
control subjects 51, 53, *53*
convenience sampling
    qualitative research 56
    quantitative research 50–1
correlation analysis 86
critical case sampling 57
cross-sectional studies 43

data collection 86–8, *87, 88*, 119–26
    coding of variables 119, 121
    directly from participants 124–6, *125*
    forms 119, *120*
    missing information 121–2
    security 123
    use of computers in 122–3
data extraction 53
data storage 85
data synthesis 31–2
demographic data 63
discussion of results 153, *154, 155*, 164–7, *164–7*
dissertation 168–9
documentation
    consent form 105–9
    data collection forms 119, *120*
    recruitment 114–15, *115*
    research protocol 89–93, *89, 90, 91*
drop-outs 129–30, *130*

ecological studies 43
EndNote 28
equipment, cost of 95
ethical review 100–5, *102–4*
Excel software 127
exclusions 129–30
extreme case sampling 57

figures 156–8, *156–9*
forest plot 32